Byrne's
ADVANCED TECHNIQUE
in
POOL
and
BILLIARDS

Robert Byrne

A Harvest Book
Harcourt Brace & Company
San Diego   New York   London

*The author invites corrections, suggestions and comments
from readers for use with credit in future editions.
Address all correspondence as follows: Robert Byrne
(Author — Please Forward), c/o Harcourt Brace & Company,
525 B Street, San Diego, CA 92101.*

Requests for permission to make copies
of any part of the work should be mailed to:
Permissions Department,
Harcourt Brace & Company, 6277 Sea Harbor Drive,
Orlando, Florida 32887-6777.

The pencil sketches in "Part Three: The Players and Their World"
were drawn by Cynthia Nelms and are based, in part, on
photographs from the following sources: Danny McGoorty — the
Byrne Collection, photo by John Grissim; James Coburn —
Billiards Digest, July 1979; Steve Mizerak — "How to Shoot Pool,
Talk Fast, and Just Plain Show Off," Miller Brewing Company,
1979; Michael Shamos — *Billiards Digest*, April 1988, photo by
David Aschkenas; Masako Katsura — the Byrne Collection, Cal-
Pictures, 1952; Raymond Ceulemans — *Billiards Digest*, August
1986, photo by Mike Panozzo; Avelino Rico — *Billiards Digest*,
August 1986, photo by Jeff Scheid; Torbjörn Blomdahl —
Billiards Digest, August 1986, photo by Jeff Scheid; Steve
Davis — *Billiards Digest*, October 1984, photo by Dave Muscroft
courtesy of *Snooker Scene*; Alex Higgins — "World Snooker with
Jack Karnehm, No. 2," *Pelham Publishing*, 1982, photo by Dave
Muscroft.

Library of Congress Cataloging-in-Publication Data
Byrne, Robert, 1930–
[Advanced technique in pool and billiards]
Byrne's advanced technique in pool and billiards/Robert Byrne.
p.   cm.
ISBN 0-15-115222-5
ISBN 0-15-614971-0 (pbk.)
1. Pool (Game)   2. Billiards.   I. Title.
II. Title: Advanced technique in pool and billiards.
GV891.B95   1990
794.7'3' — dc20   89-48204

Printed in the United States of America

First Harvest edition 1990

E F G H I

*For Mort Luby
and Mike Panozzo,
who publish a great magazine*

Contents

Part Two
BILLIARDS

Part Three

THE PLAYERS AND THEIR WORLD

Introduction

I'VE ALWAYS ENVIED—BY WHICH I MEAN HATED—NEWS-paper writers who could throw a bunch of columns together and become instant book authors. Such a deal! No need to slave for a year in the kitchen to come up with an original soufflé; just pop some leftovers in the microwave.

Now here I am myself serving up a predigested meal, namely, a selection of my articles and features from *Billiards Digest* magazine dating back to its inception in 1978.

I'm not red-faced about it at all. In fact, I'm pleased as punch, as Hubert Humphrey used to say, and I feel morally superior to the average recycler. For one thing, the articles were planned from the beginning to be chapters in a book. In the magazine I was able to write about the game in more technical detail than I could in a general book of instruction like *Byrne's Standard Book of Pool and Billiards*, which also first appeared in 1978. In that book, which was designed as a how-to-play manual aimed partly at beginners, there was no room for personality profiles, background features, or explorations of physics.

For another thing, relatively few people saw the articles when they were published, and students of the game today would have a hard time collecting them. In its early years, *Billiards Digest* had fewer than 10,000 subscribers and was not sold at newsstands. Compare 10,000 magazine subscribers to the 30 million people surveys show now play at least an occasional game of pool or billiards. There are a lot of people ready for something that goes beyond chalking the tip and drawing the ball.

More editing, updating, and rearranging was needed than I first thought to turn my journalism into a book. A lot was left behind that was ephemeral, argumentative, fuzzy, or repetitious. Articles on the same topic were combined into single chapters. Photographs that appeared with the features (Part Three) were replaced with pencil renderings by artist Cynthia Nelms. Diagrams were renumbered from 1 to 183 and keyed to the text. The goal was to create an essentially new work, one that didn't overlap my other books in any significant way and didn't have the creaky joints of the typical anthology.

Among the repetitions that were pared down were references to Robert Jewett, Ph.D., former national intercollegiate pool champion and now a research scientist with Hewlett-Packard. Most of what I know about the physics of the game I learned—and continue to learn—from him. The misconceptions he has swept from my mind over the years would fill a book as large as this. Thank you, Bob.

While the book is aimed mainly at experienced players, there is plenty here for neophytes as well. Understanding the science and the subtleties won't hurt you even if you can't yet apply the knowledge to your game. At the very least, knowing how the laws of nature apply to pool and billiard balls will help you avoid false theories, phony "systems," and teachers who talk nonsense.

Byrne's Advanced Technique isn't only about advanced technique, despite the title. It's also about why the game is so fascinating, why its tournaments are so entertaining, and why its characters are so colorful. Parts of the book even your grandmother might like.

There are dangers involved, though, in letting her (granny) read it unless she can handle a cue fairly well. The chapters on massé shots and jump shots, to take two examples, could lead to disaster, embarrassment, and loss of funds. Then, too, players who rely on instinct rather than analysis (maybe including granny) might be thrown off by learning about the physics of the game, at least initially. But it's hard to get anywhere unless you take a few chances, which goes for readers as well as writers. Tell the old girl all you know, I say, and turn her loose.

My career as a billiard journalist started in 1963 when Earl Newby, a billiard room owner in Philadelphia, started mailing out (publishing seems too grand a term) a small newspaper on the game. Newby was a sweetheart of a man, but he had no background in writing or editing and was—how shall I put this?—indifferent to the fine points of the English language. His early issues were fountains of typographical errors, misspellings, and syntactical muddles. I used to look at them in awe, wondering if a bomb had gone off in the printing plant.

Once I sent him an account of a California tournament along with a handwritten cover note that read: "Dear Earl, Here's something you and your readers may be interested in." When the paper came in the mail a month or so later, I leafed through the chaos until I found my article and saw with dismay that the first sentence was: "Dear Earl, Here's something you and your readers may be interested in."

But for years nobody else could see that the industry needed a publication or had the energy and nerve to start one. He didn't let his lack of technical qualifications stop him. (A lesson for us all.) He provided a way for players, tournament promoters, manufacturers, dealers, wholesalers, and just plain fans to communicate with each other and find out what was going on. I salute him. He would be amazed to see how many billiard publications there are now; almost every tavern league has at least a newsletter.

In about 1970 I switched my allegiance to *The National Bowlers Journal and Billiard Review* because—*mirabile dictu!*—the editor paid for freelance contributions. Writers have to eat just like people who work for a living.

In 1978 *Bowlers Journal* spun off the handsome, professionally edited *Billiards Digest*, from whose pages this book is drawn. For the first time in history, pool fans could open a magazine and see photos of players, equipment, and rooms in full color. The first issue of *BD* had 64 pages; a dozen years later it was almost twice as big. (For a subscription call 1-312-266-7171.) The magazine's growth reflects the growth in the game over the same period.

Pool is in boom times, make no mistake about it. New rooms, especially of the upscale variety, are opening everywhere, and tournaments of all kinds are growing in terms of entrants, spectators, and prize funds. A Gallup survey shows that there are as many pool players as joggers, a fact that surprises people who have never had to swerve to avoid a pool player. The advertising industry suddenly loves pool. Pool is in. Pool is chic.

Television networks, though, with the partial exception of ESPN, have yet to notice how the recreational landscape has changed. When they do, there is no telling what dizzying heights the game will attain.

Robert Byrne
Mill Valley, Calif.

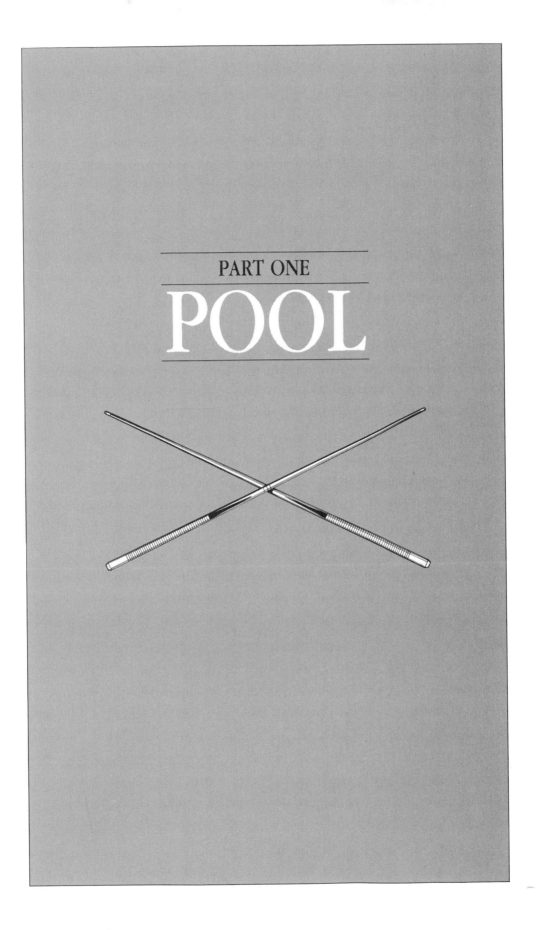

PART ONE
POOL

The Fundamentals—Facts and Fantasies

What is the poor student of the game supposed to do when the experts contradict themselves and each other, not just on advanced strategy but on fundamentals? One would think that after 200 years there would be agreement on how to stand and how to hold and use a cue, but such is not the case. Players can't even agree on what type and size of cue to use.

If you are trying to improve your game, remember these facts: Not all good players are good teachers; some good players are wrong on how they get the results they do; what works for any given good player may not work for you; and just because a statement is made by a good player or authority doesn't necessarily mean it is true.

In other words, take even what *I* say with a grain of salt. You have to develop your own style of play, which means finding out what works best for you. The point is so obvious it seems unnecessary to state it. Watch 50 top players in a tournament and you will see a wide variety of postures, grips, and strokes, yet teachers and writers continue to say that the student should stand and hold the cue in a certain way and use a certain kind of stroke. Nonsense!

The stance. Forget all that stuff about facing the shot with your hand at your hip, taking a half-step forward, turning 45 degrees, etc. Stand any way you want to, provided you feel comfortable and one eye is over the cue. If you have to be told to put one eye over the cue, you are a hopeless case and should stick to bowling. Some good players bend slightly at the knees, some keep the legs straight and spread their feet wide apart; some balance their weight evenly, some put more on the forward foot; some put quite a bit of weight on the bridge hand, some hardly any; some turn almost sideways, some face the shot more squarely. What should you do? Whatever feels right. There is no *correct* way to stand.

Notice, though, that all the snooker professionals, who play a game where accuracy of hit is all-important, lean down so far that their chins are on the cue. The three-cushion champions, on the other hand, who are more concerned with carom and rebound angles, stand up straighter. That observation leads me to think that pool players who need a precise hit should crouch low and aim the cue like a rifle, the way the snooker players do. Missing shots you normally make? Are you in a slump? Try leaning down more. Because of laziness or fatigue, players sometimes don't bend over as much as they should.

The bridge. All you have to do is provide a support for the cue that enables it to move back and forth without wobbling from side to side. It is up to you to find a comfortable way to hold your fingers. Only when you are shooting hard or using a lot of sidespin is it necessary to form a "looped" bridge. On most shots an open or V bridge is sufficient and even an advantage because the entire shaft is visible for aiming. Harry Sims has a snug, solid, looped bridge, but his fingers spring open at the moment of impact—that would have to be considered a flaw and it is something you wouldn't teach a student—but it didn't stop him from twice winning the national billiard championship.

The grip. Should there be a space between the cue and your fingers? Should you hold it with just two fingers or all five? Should the wrist be loose or locked? People write and phone to ask me such questions. Hold the cue any way that feels right to you and ignore all other advice, including mine. Florida's Carlos Hallon, the brilliant three-cushion player, holds his cue at the tips of his thumb and forefinger, the way Queen Victoria held a teacup, yet he can slam the balls with sledgehammer force if he has to. California's Jim McFarlane, a terror when he was known as Whitey the Beer Salesman, always holds the cue at the extreme rear, which doesn't mean he can't take your money. A sprinkling of great pool and billiard players, Al Gilbert among them, use a slip stroke, in which the hand takes a new grip just before the trigger is pulled. Some players have a flexible or even a "whippy" wrist, while others keep it rigid. A guy in Kentucky wrote to ask if I had ever experimented with "the reverse slip stroke," in which the cue is more or less thrown into the cueball. The answer is no.

What all this suggests to me is that the grip isn't as important as it has been made out to be. All kinds of grips can be made to work.

The stroke. A lot of mythology surrounds the stroke. Some players believe that uncanny, mystical effects are possible with one kind of stroke or another. A loose wrist, it has been claimed, will make the cueball do one thing, while a locked wrist on the same shot will make it do another. Not true. A long follow-through does one thing, a check stroke another. False. Use a tight grip here, a loose grip there, stroke with the wrist here, with the shoulder there, twist the wrist here, swerve the cue there. Spare me!

Here are the facts, and I wouldn't lie to you on something so important. In the physics formulas that describe the motion of balls and the collisions between them, there are no coefficients or factors for wrists, grips, or strokes. They aren't needed. The cueball moves down the table with a certain speed, spin, and direction, which can be applied to it with almost any kind of stroke or grip. The cueball doesn't care what you are thinking about when you hit it, or whether or not your wrist is tight or relaxed—all it "knows" is where the tip hits it and how hard. Whether or not you twist the cue or check your stroke or lock your wrist or follow through makes no difference to the cueball at all.

Consider the follow-through. The contact between the tip and the cueball is almost instantaneous. Once the cueball leaves the tip, it doesn't care what you do with the cue. When the instant of contact has passed, you no longer have any control over the cueball. The only reason for teaching students to follow straight through the cueball is because it helps them *deliver* the cue into the ball properly. Once they know how to hit the ball it no longer matters if they follow through or not.

But there is no particular reason why you *shouldn't* follow through, unless there are balls to be avoided. Once the cue is moving forward it is a waste of energy to bring it to a sudden stop.

You can make quick warm-up strokes or slow; you can pause at the rear of the final backswing or not. As in the other fundamentals, you have a wide range of acceptable styles to choose from. Find what is right for you and don't let a teacher try to make you his clone.

What really counts. While good fundamentals and basic technique are undeniably important, other factors are even more important in reaching top levels. What does it take to become a champion? Here are just a few things you must have: steady nerves; good eyesight; good hand-eye coordination; enough intelligence to learn how best to analyze an array of balls; a good memory so that you can learn from your mistakes; a knack for knowing when to attack and when to defend (which means being able to estimate percentages on every shot); a relentless lust for competition; so much desire to improve that you wake up in the morning thinking of shots and moves; a will to win so strong that a defeat gnaws at you for hours or days; the ability to concentrate while aiming (instead of just going through the motions of aiming); the discipline to practice with intensity; a willingness to put everything else in life second—especially when you are still a teenager; and an imagination that enables you to come up with creative solutions to problems you've never seen before.

Once you reach the top level, you can relax a little and turn some of your attention to trivialities like family and career. Getting there, though, takes a terrific investment of time and attention. It takes far more than changing cues or finding a new way to hold your wrist.

Some of the ingredients, like eyes, nerves, coordination, intelligence, and imagination, are part of the package you were born with and can't be improved with teaching or practice. Sorry.

My aim regarding fundamentals is to encourage you to develop your own style without slavishly aping a teacher. A student complains: "I can't believe you think the stroke is unimportant." Please! A good stroke is absolutely essential, that much is clear even to me. What isn't clear is what constitutes a good stroke. Should you adopt the pump-handle, teeter-totter style of Efren Reyes? The free-flowing classic style of Ralph Greenleaf? The slip-stroke of Ray Kilgore or Al Gilbert? The solid compactness of Raymond Ceulemans? The slow, deliberate approach of Bud Harris? The precious side-arm of the young Willie Hoppe?

With such a smorgasbord of styles to choose from, it is impossible to say which is best for any particular player. All that is necessary for top-flight play is the ability to hit the cueball at precisely the right spot, in precisely the right direction, with precisely the right speed. How you do it is up to you. I would like to be able to say that one thing all good strokes have in common is an absence of wobbling or veering during the warm-ups and final delivery, but there are even exceptions to that. I knew one superb hustler who worked on making his stroke crooked. Some hustlers, to make themselves look lucky rather than good, always address the cueball in the center, applying the necessary English only at the moment of contact, which requires veering on the approach. (That dodge may have been used by Jack Carr, thought to be the discoverer of sidespin, in England in the early years of the last century. See *Roberts on Billiards,* by John Roberts, 1869, page 68.)

How, an anguished reader asks, does Mike Massey jump his cueball entirely over a ball and still draw back the length of the table? What is his mechanical secret? The secret is called talent. He has a gift for hitting the cueball off center with both precision and explosive power, along with the knowledge of what is required on the shot and the hand-eye coordination to achieve it. Things like these are sometimes lumped together under the heading "touch." There are a thousand mechanical secrets that a player can learn, but touch, talent, and genius are built-in features.

Let's explode some other myths. Practically every top player will tell you that if you spin a ball in place like a top and then knock it slowly down the table with another ball, it will curve toward the direction of the spin— that is, right English will make a ball curve to the right, right? Wrong! A massé effect is needed to make a ball curve. Try it. If you don't have the digital dexterity to spin a ball in place with your fingers, shoot a stop shot with heavy English. When you roll another ball into the spinning ball, it will take off at an odd angle because of throw, then it will roll in a straight line (on clean, unpitted cloth). Knowing this has great practical use. If you are using a perfectly level cue, and you are applying middle-ball sidespin to the cueball, you don't have to allow for curve. Only when you are shooting slightly down on the cueball will it curve.

Bob Jewett has a trick way of making a cueball curve to the left even though it has right-hand spin. It is a proposition bet that may be unknown even to Willie Jopling, a collector of them. Put a cube of chalk mouth-side-up on the rail and rest the cueball on it. Drop to one knee and shoot into the cueball from below, angling the cue at an upward angle of 30 or 40 degrees. If you hit the ball right of center it will take a left curve as it goes down the table.

Some players apparently think that some sort of English or other can cause an object ball to go all the way into a pocket and jump back out onto the table. No way. When that happens it is because of stupid pocket design. One would think that after hundreds of years of experience the industry could make pockets that would retain balls no matter how hard they are hit, but such is not the case. Of course, even with a perfect pocket, it will always be possible to send a ball into it several inches off the table so that it strikes the upper rim and bounces back, but I'm not complaining about that. If you still think English has something to do with it, place a cueball in front of a pocket that sometimes spits back balls, and shoot the cueball straight in with various kinds of spin. The spin will have little or no effect on the ratio of rejection. The effect will definitely be zero if an object ball is used, because only a very small fraction of spin can be transferred from ball to ball.

Can a ball be made to hug the rail? Not an object ball, unless there is a groove in the cloth or the table isn't level. An object ball will *stay* on the rail, of course, if hit accurately . . . and maybe it will appear to hug the rail. A cueball can be made to hug the rail by elevating the butt of the cue and imparting massé action, but that kind of spin can't be transferred to an object ball.

Can more English be put on a cueball with a small tip or a large one? In the range of sizes that is practical, from 11 mm. to 13 mm., it doesn't make any difference. I think it is a little easier to hit the cueball exactly where you want to with the smaller size, but a tiny tip usually means a shaft that is too flimsy and a tip that will wear out too fast. (If anybody cares, my own tip is 12 mm. My cue weighs 18.75 ounces and has shafts with the stiff European taper. In my opinion, almost all American pool cues have shafts that are too flexible.)

Is a loose wrist the key to lively draw action? No. What you need is a well-chalked cue and a very low hit.

Transferring Spin from Ball to Ball

Can English on the cueball help an object ball into a pocket, or keep it out? No. A spinning ball rolling so slowly that it just barely touches one side of a pocket may drop or stay up depending on the direction of the spin, but you can't control speed that accurately under game conditions, and you can't deliberately put enough spin on an object ball to matter. It is possible to make a cueball scratch in the side when approaching from a shadow angle by using slow speed and a lot of spin, but I can't think of a practical application outside of proposition bets. Forget trying to assist the object ball into the pocket by transferring spin to it from the cueball—you will only make it more difficult to get an accurate hit.

Consider shot A in Diagram 1. There is nothing you can do in terms of English on the cueball that will "help" the object ball into the corner pocket.

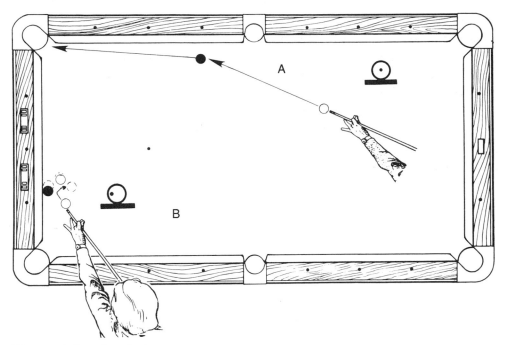

Diagram 1. Transfer of spin

If this is game ball and there is no need to play position, the best course is a center-ball hit on the cueball, a level cue, and as accurate a hit as possible on the object ball. Any use of spin on the cueball makes the shot tougher.

It is true that left English will put a little right English on the object ball, but with soft or medium speed the transferred spin lasts only a few inches; by the time the object ball reaches the corner pocket it will be rolling naturally. (Try it and see—the object ball will not be spinning when it reaches the corner no matter what you put on the cueball. Even with great speed—ridiculous for this shot—the ball will not be turning enough to see or matter. Banks, though, are different.) Further, the left English will make the object ball "throw" slightly off line to the right, making it harder to determine the correct aiming point. If your cue isn't exactly level, left English will make the cueball curve to the left on its way to the ball, and if you use any speed you have "squirt" to contend with as well. (Squirt is what I call the way the cueball diverges in the direction opposite the English.)

We have all seen spinning object balls go into pockets because the spin carries them in off-the-jaw, but that is always after the ball has hit other balls. The only way to get heavy spin on an object ball is to carom it off other balls. You can't get meaningful "into-the-pocket" spin on an object ball by putting the opposite spin on the cueball, and to try to do it at the expense of accuracy is crazy.

English, or "side," as the English put it, makes it harder to pocket the object ball. Ask any English snooker player. Snooker is played on a 6-by-12 table with narrow pockets and demands such extreme accuracy that very little sidespin is used. It is a game of follow, draw, and dead ball strokes. Terry Griffiths, 1979 World Snooker champion, states in his book *Complete Snooker,* that he hits the cueball somewhere on its vertical axis 99 percent of the time! The lesson for American pool players is clear: Avoid sidespin whenever possible.

Maybe their unfamiliarity with sidespin is what makes so many snooker professionals deny that any spin at all can be transferred to the object ball. Current world champion Steve Davis has written that the idea that spin can be transferred is "rubbish." John Spencer, another top snooker pro, says in his book *Spencer on Pool,* that he is asked at least once a week whether or not cueball spin has any effect on the object ball. "My opinion," he writes, "is that you can impart side to an object ball only unintentionally and not in a way that you can gain any advantage from it."

It is amazing to me that in a country where English billiards (a combination of pool and carom billiards) is still popular there should be any doubt about whether or not spin can be transferred. Of course it can, and it is easy to prove.

In shot B of Diagram 1, a rail nurse position common in straight billiards as well as English billiards, the correct shot is a soft kissback off the red ball. (Note the short bridge.) Left sidespin on the cueball will cause the red ball to move toward the white ball, keeping the two object balls close together for another easy shot. Kissing back off the red without cueball spin, or with right spin, will freeze the red ball in position or make it move to the left, *away* from the white ball. This is simple and indisputable proof that spin can be transferred.

Another easy proof is to put an object ball on the head spot and drive it across the foot spot into the exact center of the end rail using firm speed and heavy sidespin on the cueball, as in Diagram 2. (This is not easy to do because the object ball will be thrown off line by the cueball spin, which requires compensation.) If you shoot hard enough and with enough cueball spin, the object ball will rebound at somewhat of an angle because of the slight turn ("spin" seems too strong a word) it will have picked up from the cueball. Influencing the rebound of an object ball in this way is very important in making off-angle banks in pool and in making "gather" shots in straight billiards and balkline. (In snooker, the margin of error is so small that players normally play safe rather than trying to influence banks with spin.)

There is a way to demonstrate transfer of spin directly. A slick surface, like glass or plastic, is best. Set up a cueball and two object balls in a straight line, as shown at the top of Diagram 3. Using heavy sidespin and a hard stroke, drive the first object ball so squarely into the second one that it stops dead, which is harder than it looks. When this is done correctly, the first

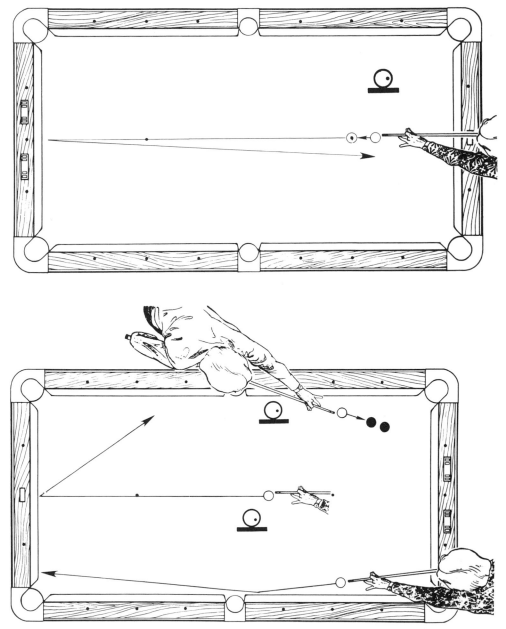

Diagrams 2 and 3: Transfer of spin

object ball can sometimes be seen rotating several times before coming to rest.

The amount of sidespin that can be transmitted from one ball to another is quite small, about two percent, and can be ignored when considering a second object ball. In the above example, you can add a third object ball to stop the second one—you will never see the second one turning after the collisions.

The phenomenon of English transfer is especially important on bank shots, and the closer to a right angle the bank is, the more pronounced is the effect. If you shoot a cueball straight into a rail, sidespin affects the rebound angle tremendously. The middle of Diagram 3 shows what can be done with maximum right spin. (Hit the cueball slightly below center and softly for the greatest effect.) At the bottom of the diagram, the cueball approaches the rail at a small angle; here the rebound angle will be almost identical no matter which side of the cueball is struck.

It follows that transfer of English will be of most importance on a shot that involves an almost perpendicular approach to a rail. Such a shot is given in Diagram 4. At the top, the cueball is about six inches from the object ball. Assume that the paths to the obvious pockets are blocked by other balls, or assume that the game is one-pocket and you must make the ball in the upper right-hand corner. The shot can be played as a bank. Use heavy left English and enough right English will be imparted to the object ball to affect its rebound as shown. In fact, in a position like this you can easily transfer too much English.

At the bottom of Diagram 4 is the shot as it is usually presented. Here, enough sidespin is put on the object ball simply by the way the cueball rubs across its face. It is essential not to use any left-hand English on the cueball at this angle because it would cause the cueball to roll across the face of the object ball and would give the object ball no sidespin.

It has been alleged by at least one expert that the position at the bottom of Diagram 4 should be approached with an elevated cue so that the cueball leaves the cloth and gives the object ball a downward blow. This, it was claimed, will impart a massé effect to the object ball and make it curve

Diagram 4. Transfer of spin

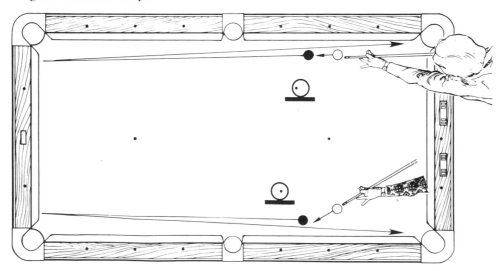

slightly to the left. I deny that an object ball can be made to curve in any significant or practical manner by means of a jumping cueball. The friction between the balls isn't great enough for the massé effect to take place. Even trying to make the *cueball* curve is almost impossible without a well-chalked tip—think how much less friction there is between two balls.

Which is not to say that interference can't be avoided by getting the object ball airborne. Imagine a straight-in shot similar to the one at the top of Diagram 4, and imagine that there is a ball a foot away from the object ball that just barely blocks the path to the pocket. A player might consider elevating his cue to make the cueball hit the first ball slightly from above with the hope that the object ball would then jump over the edge of the interfering ball. A well-known exhibition shot is to make the cueball jump over a cue placed on the table and strike an object ball that in turn jumps over a cue before going into the pocket. Not terribly difficult. (See page 126 of *Byrne's Treasury of Trick Shots in Pool and Billiards.*)

Which brings us to Diagram 5 and the trick shot that for some reason is one of the best known in the world. Yet it's not easy to make all four balls. The ball that's hard to make is the one that has to bank the length of the table. If you've read this far you know that you have to give it a little right spin, either by using heavy left on the cueball or by placing the cueball at the start so that it crosses the ball from left to right. Aim directly between the two middle balls so that the end ball is given enough speed to reach the opposite side pocket. There's a final point to consider: If the balls are dirty, it may be unnecessary to do anything with the cueball; the ball to be banked may pick up enough sidespin as it leaves the end ball.

Diagram 5. Transfer of spin

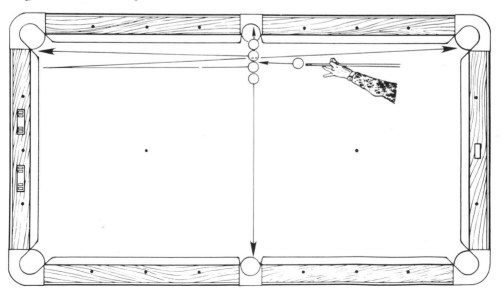

Four Sidespin Falsehoods

Consider the following four falsehoods:

1. After hitting an object ball on a cut shot, a cueball with sidespin will move forward more slowly than one without sidespin.
2. Sidespin affects the direction the cueball takes off the object ball.
3. A cueball with sidespin divides a cluster better than one without spin.
4. Sidespin on a cueball increases when the cueball hits an object ball.

I'll take up the points in order.

1. On a cut shot, what determines the cueball's speed after contact depends on the cueball's initial linear speed, the amount of the cut, and the amount of topspin or backspin. Sidespin has nothing to do with it. Sidespin becomes significant when the cueball touches a rail—then it influences both the speed and the rebound angle off the rail.
2. Sidespin has no significant effect on the direction the cueball takes off an object ball on a cut shot. At impact, the cueball path changes to the right-angle (or tangent) line, which is 90 degrees from the path taken by the object ball. Sidespin has no effect, but topspin and backspin do. If the cueball has topspin, then it will bend forward from the right angle along a parabolic curve; with backspin it will curve in the opposite direction. The curves are shown on pages 54, 56, 70, and 71 in *Byrne's Standard Book of Pool and Billiards* and can be seen being traced in slow motion in Volume II of *Byrne's Standard Video of Pool.*
3. Urging players to use sidespin when sending the cueball into a pack or cluster is poor advice. The cueball won't wade in like Hulk Hogan and throw balls in all directions because it is spinning; the speed of the object balls leaving the cluster depends entirely on the linear speed of the cueball when it hits the cluster and the point of contact.

   Topspin, though, is necessary if you need to make the cueball burrow through the cluster.

   There are other reasons for not advocating sidespin on primary or secondary break shots. Sidespin raises the problems of squirt (deflection), curve, and object-ball throw as well as increasing the chance of a miscue. If sidespin *did* help in dividing a pack, then nine-ball players would use it on the break.

   Splitting clusters often decides the game, and because with a large pack considerable force must be used, accuracy goes down. Don't add to the chance of missing by using sidespin, which doesn't help in any event.

   Some bowlers think that "a working ball," by which they mean a ball that has sidespin, throws the pins around more energetically, but they are wrong. A bowling ball curves only while it is sliding on the lane;

once it starts to roll it travels in a straight line. It is the changed angle of attack on the pins that makes the difference. (See *Sports Science, Physical Laws and Optimum Performance,* by Peter J. Brancazio, Simon and Schuster, 1984, pages 99 and 100.)

4. It's okay to say the sun comes up and the sun goes down provided you know that in fact the sun stays put while the earth moves. It's not accurate to say that cueball spin increases when the cueball hits an object ball, though that's how it looks. What *really* happens is that the impact between the balls reduces the linear speed of the cueball while the sidespin remains the same. When you use heavy sidespin and hit an object ball full, the spin you see is merely what the cue tip put on the cueball in the first place, not something mysterious that arose because of the impact.

When a cueball hits an object ball full in the face, for all practical purposes it stops dead and all of the linear speed is transferred to the object ball. What the cueball does next depends on whether or not it has topspin or backspin. It if slid into the object ball, it stays put (the stop shot). If it had topspin, even the topspin imparted by the natural forward roll, then it will follow forward as the spin grabs the cloth. Backspin makes the cueball back up. The slight hesitation before the follow and draw take effect can be seen if you watch carefully.

On the left side of Diagram 6, the idea is to get good position of the 2-ball for a break in a game of straight pool. Follow will send the cueball along a path to point A, depending on the force of the hit. Adding some right English will change the angle off the first rail, sending the ball to B, or thereabouts, not so far down the table. (Note how the cueball starts out

Diagram 6. Effects of sidespin

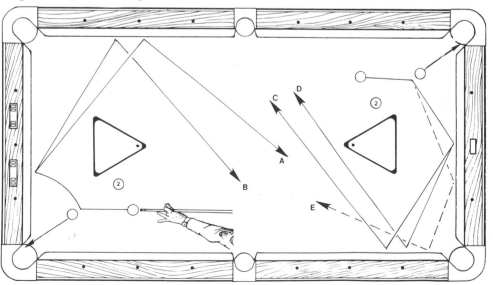

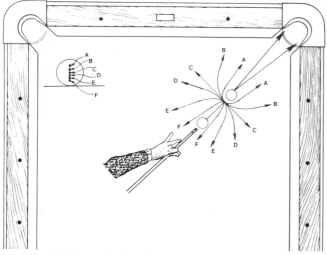

Diagram 7. Effects of sidespin

along the right-angle line off the object ball, then bends forward.)

On the right side of the diagram is the same position. Using slide instead of follow keeps the cueball on the right-angle line off the object ball, sending it along the diagrammed path to point C, or nearby. Adding sidespin changes the rebound off the first rail as shown by the path that ends at D. On a fuller hit, which would take more of the speed of the cueball, the cueball may still be spinning strongly when it hits the second rail, sending it to the vicinity of E. Spin off the second (and third) rail is action familiar to every three-cushion player and can be achieved only with hits fuller than half-ball (approximately).

Diagram 7 shows what is possible with varying amounts of topspin and backspin. By sending the object ball into one part of the pocket or another and by varying the hit on the vertical axis (sidespin is immaterial), it is possible to make the cueball move away in any direction. Some of the angles are hard to achieve consistently. At the left is a player's-eye view of the cueball showing point of tip contact.

The Best Ways to Practice

Students of the game who are trying to improve usually spend too much time pocketing balls and not enough time on position. Controlling the cueball is the key to success, yet there are few practice drills that zero in on position play alone.

Despite the obvious value of working on drills, most players dislike them because of the dullness and repetition. Practicing by yourself, in fact, can do more harm than good. Lacking the motivation to try your best on every shot, you can easily get careless and end up merely reinforcing the flaws in your game. Competition is the key. Ever notice that almost every top player learned his skills at a public room rather than at home or in a club?

In *Byrne's Standard Book* there are ten position practice shots presented in the form of a game in an effort to avoid boredom. Following are a few more that will challenge both beginners and professionals.

In all of the shots, making the object ball is easy; the challenge is to control the cueball with as much precision as possible. Practice against a friend or an enemy. He gets three tries, you get three tries, and whoever comes the closest to the goal wins. Put some money on it so you'll stay alert.

At the top of Diagram 8 the object ball is at A and the cueball is at B. The first test is to shoot a stop shot, allowing the cueball to drift no more than the width of a piece of chalk, with the cueball at B, C, D, and E. A useful thing to learn here is that a stop shot can be done either with a firm stroke and a middle ball hit or with a soft stroke and a very low hit. Of course the farther you are from the object ball the more speed is needed.

Next, with the object ball at A and the cueball at B, draw the cueball to B, to C, to D, and to E. Leaving the object ball at A, start with the cueball at C and try drawing it to points B, C, D, and E. If you are an advanced player, you can try starting with the cueball at D and E. Getting draw action with the object ball at A and cueball at E takes very good technique.

If you are competing against someone, use a coin to mark the final position of the cueball.

At the bottom of Diagram 8 is a series of shots designed to enhance

Diagram 8. Practice methods

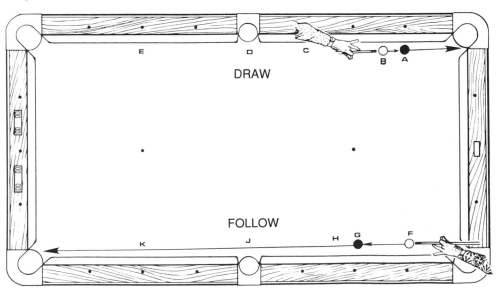

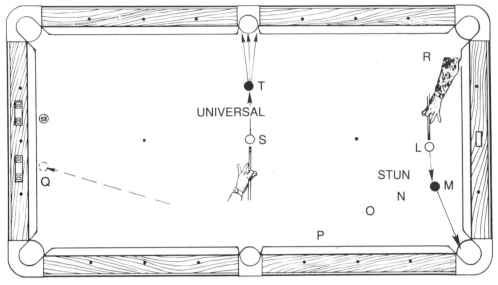

Diagram 9. Practice methods

your judgment of follow. The cueball is always placed at F to start. With the object ball at G, make it in the corner and try to leave the cueball at H, J, and K. It is possible to leave the cueball at H by shooting very softly, but you should also be able to do it using a lot of speed, hitting the cueball just slightly above center. With the object ball at J, follow to K.

It is easier to judge the length of the cueball's roll on follow shots than draw shots, a good thing to remember in nine ball when you have ball in hand.

It is absolutely essential to have command of the so-called stun shot, also called the dead-ball draw. It takes a certain touch. The idea is to make the cueball slide into the object ball with neither topspin or backspin; the result is that the cueball will then drift along the tangent line from the collision point. Again, it can be accomplished either with a firm stroke and a middle ball hit, or a softer stroke and a low hit. (When the shot is straight in, the cueball will stop dead, as in a stop shot.)

Study Diagram 9. With the cueball at L and the object ball at M, you should be able to pocket the object ball and make the cueball die at N or O or P, and you should be able to do it with fairly good precision. From the same starting position, you can use a harder stroke and a little right English to make the cueball end up at the other end of the table at Q for an easy shot at the 9-ball. Pretty easy when you get used to it, but can you leave the cueball at N, O, P, and Q when the cueball is farther away, at R? Success on this drill requires a good feel for the relationship between speed and distance.

In the middle of Diagram 9 is what I call the Universal Position Shot. The cueball is in the exact center of the table and the object ball is one diamond away from the side pocket. From that position, through the use of varying speeds, spins, and hits (you can cheat the pocket as shown), it is possible to make the ball and send the cueball *to any point on the table*. Try it with a friend. Put a coin anywhere on the table and see how close you can come to it with the cueball in three chances. Then he has his turn. Mark the cueball stopping points with a damp finger.

I'd like to see a competition with shots like these among the top players, perhaps as a special feature at a tournament. It would sort out the shotmakers from the position players and it would demonstrate why it is that the pros get so many easy shots.

How to Teach Position Play

We all know players—maybe members of a local bar league team, maybe somebody who shows up at the billiard room only occasionally—who haven't yet realized that thinking ahead is often just as important as pocketing the ball. Some are fairly good shotmakers and have been playing socially for years, yet rarely put together a decent run. How can you get them to pay more attention to cueball control? The examples in this section will help because they lead to immediate results. (I assume you know a pastime player who is willing to learn and listen; not all are.)

Place the 4, 5, and 8 as shown in Diagram 10. Position the cueball exactly between the 4 and 5. There are thousands upon thousands of social players who have trouble ending a game of eight ball from this position

Diagram 10. Position play

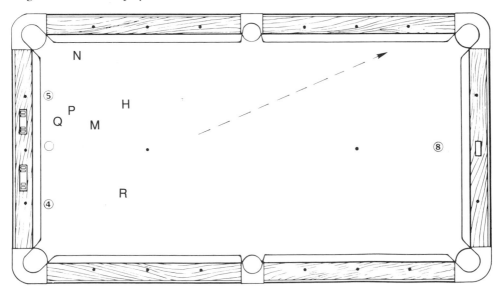

Before doing any teaching, see how many times your student can do it in, say, five tries.

The key, of course, is getting an angle on the second ball, which depends on the ability to put a little follow or draw on the cueball, skills you might have to teach some students. If the 5 is a little farther from the rail than the cueball, or if the pockets are "easy," draw the cueball to M, from which point it is easy to cut in the 4 and send the cueball along the dashed line to position on the 8. Once the student can do it, block the pattern with a ball at P. Now what? Follow to N and out to H.

A good method of teaching the value of advance planning is to set up several balls and hand the cueball to the student for placement, which is advocated by Jerry Briesath of Madison, Wis., perhaps the premier teacher in the country. In Diagram 10, a good spot for the cueball is Q, from where it is easy to pocket the 5 and bring the cueball to M for the desired angle on the 4. An additional point you can make with this diagram, if you think your student is ready for it, is that it would be better to shoot the 4 first and end up at R rather than H because the 5 is easier to reach for a right-handed player.

In Diagram 11, the challenge is to make the 6 and 7 and get the cueball to the other end of the table for the 8 (not shown). A stop-shot on the 7 is a blunder because then the 6 is straight in. A stop-shot on the 6 is good because the 7 can be cut in and the cueball sent off point W on the rail and down the table. Once the student understands, block the path with a ball at S. Now a way out is to shoot the 7 and follow to point T, which provides an angle on the 6. And if a ball at U interferes? Shoot the 7 first and draw the cueball to V. The use of draw to avoid a straight-in shot, it depresses me to report, is a novel concept to many.

Diagram 12 shows a 7-ball near the side and the 8 at the left end. After placing the balls, hand the student the cueball and ask where he would put it to run out a game of eight ball. Is the problem too simple? No. Try it on players not accustomed to thinking ahead and you'll see. Probably the safest plan in Diagram 12 is to place the cueball at K and send the cueball on the indicated path. If that path is blocked, the cueball can be put at H and sent to M with follow. And if that can't be done because of the opponent's balls, the cueball can be put at P and sent three or four rails to the area around M (part of the path is shown by dashed lines). Prediction: the first time your student tries the latter path, he will hit the 7 too full.

The position in Diagram 13 arose in a professional tournament at the Jointed Cue in Sacramento. A very fine player had ball in hand. The 4 was near the corner pocket and the 5 was at the other end of the table (out of the diagram). Perhaps because of tournament pressure (it's easy to think clearly in the bleachers), he failed to think of putting the cueball on the lip of the pocket and playing the 4 in the other corner pocket. The position

Diagrams 11, 12, and 13: Position play

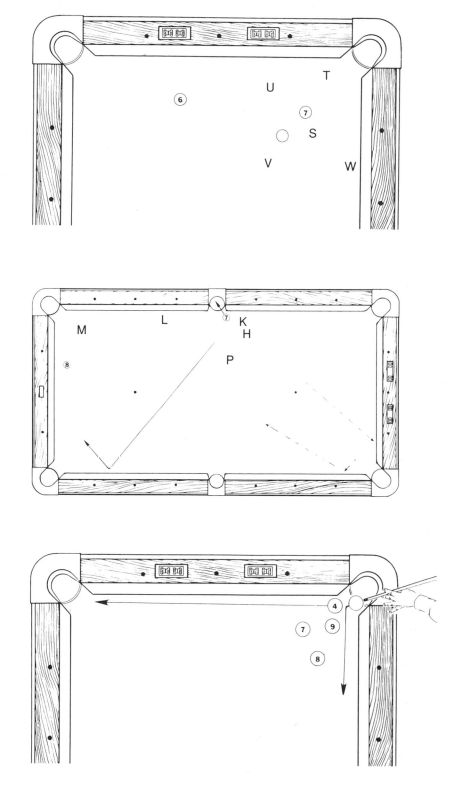

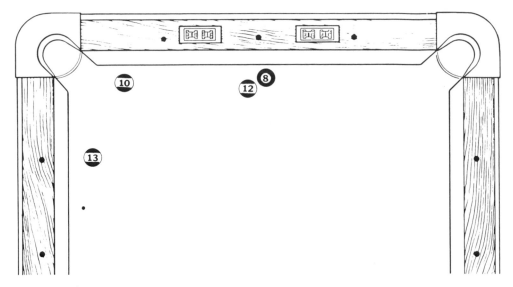

Diagram 14. Position play

can be used as a challenge with fairly good players. Jump shots can be blocked with extra balls.

Then there is the common problem of breaking up clusters. Diagram 14 is a position of heavenly simplicity. If your student had cueball in hand in a game of eight ball, would he know where to put it? (Ball in hand is typical of nine ball, but the kind of student I am thinking of tends to respond better to eight-ball examples.) The correct answer is to put the cueball on the dot shown near 13. From there the 13 can be pocketed and the 12 and 8 lightly spread. The 10 makes it easy to get position on the 12.

The point of the examples given here—and others you can make up yourself—is that pool requires thinking as much as hand-eye coordination. A little foresight often results in a series of simple shots.

How to Aim Carom Shots

To call yourself a player, you have to be able to stop the cueball dead on straight-in shots of any length. It's not easy at a distance of, say, five feet. Very often, a cueball that drifts even an inch after contact with the object ball will stop a run. If you can't stop the cueball absolutely dead, especially on short shots, practice until you can, for the technique is essential in top-class play. You can't completely kill the cueball on cuts, but you can make some great caroms with the same "stop action."

Stop action results if the cueball is sliding when it hits the object ball: no backspin and no topspin. You have to be able to make the cueball slide into the object ball over a wide range of speeds if you want to stop it dead on straight-in shots. A very low hit and soft speed will do it, as will hard speed and a hit just slightly below center. Why you have to be able to do it all ways becomes apparent when the shot isn't straight in. The position player has to be able to judge the distance the cueball will travel after the hit, which is a function of speed, and the carom player has to be able to judge the cueball's direction, which depends on the degree of cut.

If the cueball is sliding when it reaches the object ball on a cut shots, then it will travel along the "tangent line," which is the line at right angles to the line formed by the balls at the instant of contact. Another way to think of it is this: On a cut shot, if the cueball is sliding at contact, the two diverging ball paths form a right angle. (The angle is slightly less than 90 degrees because of "throw," and because balls are never perfectly elastic, but I'll ignore that to simplify the explanation.)

Some readers may wonder what happens when the cueball has topspin or backspin on cut shots. In those cases the cueball starts out along the right-angle line, then bends forward or backward. Here we'll stick to straight cueball paths, which result from zero spin.

Take the position in Diagram 15. To hit the 4-ball and make the 9 with the cueball requires finding the tangent line, driving the 1 ball at right angles to it, and hitting the cueball so that it's sliding when it contacts the 4. One way to find the tangent line is to rest the tip of your cue on the cloth at

Diagram 15. Carom shots

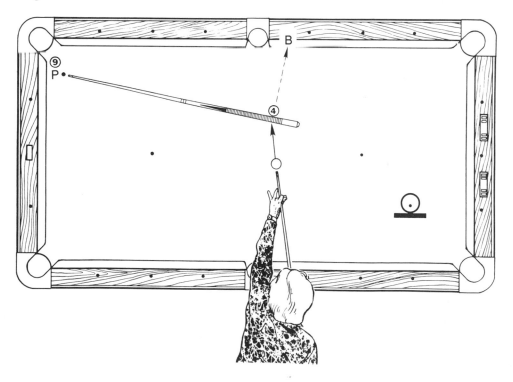

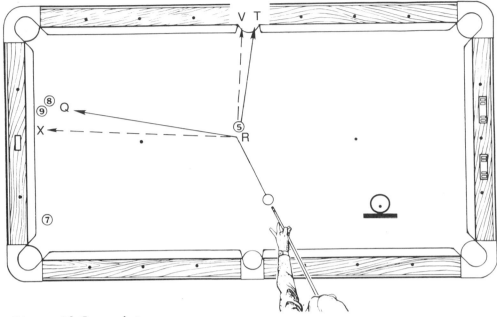

Diagram 16. Carom shots

point P, which is a point over which the cueball must pass to cut the 9 in, and pivot the butt toward the 4 until it almost touches it. The center of the cue is now the tangent line. Next, project a line through the 4 at right angles to the cue, and mentally locate point B, where the line crosses the rail. If you can drive the 4 into point B with stop action (slide) on the cueball, the carom will be successful.

In Diagram 16 the game is also nine ball. The task is to cut the 5 into the side and break up a cluster on the end rail. If the cluster is at point Q, as shown, then drive the object ball into the right side of the pocket with slide on the cueball, because QRT is a right angle. If the cluster is at X, use the left side of the pocket because XRV is a right angle. The calculation is fairly simple and is within the reach of pastime players. Master players can hit a cluster anywhere on the end rail by using various amounts of follow and draw and judging the resulting curved cueball paths.

In Diagram 17 there is a carom even weak players can make. Hit the 7-ball head on at a reasonable speed and it will carom off the 8 into the corner. In Diagram 18 the geometry is the same but several feet of distance have been added between the 7 and the 8. If you drive the 7 into the same spot on the 8, you must shoot very hard. Why? So the 7 will still be sliding when it hits the 8. If the 7 has time to pick up natural forward roll on its way to the 8, its path leaving the 8 will be curved because of the topspin and may look as drawn, which is a miss.

Note that I have changed my shirt for each diagram. That's not necessary unless you sweat a lot.

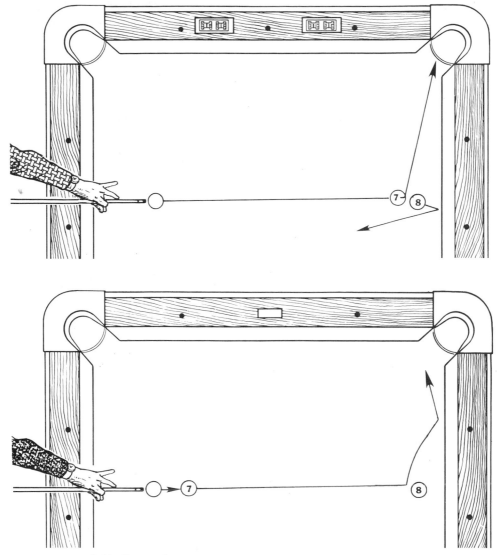

Diagrams 17 and 18: Carom shots

The Throw Effect on Cut Shots

For years I wondered why balls "throw" off the line indicated by contact points only when they are frozen or nearly so. I also wondered why beginners tend to hit object balls too thick more often than too thin. Could it be that throw is involved whenever balls collide, even on simple cut shots? Every top player I mentioned the possibility to looked at me as if I didn't have both oars in the water.

In 1981 I tested my suspicions in a systematic way. The results were startling. I think they destroy some widely held myths about the proper way to aim a cut shot. They also show that top players tend to use outside English on cut shots not for reasons of affectation but because they have learned unconsciously that they must nullify the throw effect if they want to hit the theoretical contact point and still make the shot.

My inspiration came from browsing through the excellent book *How I Play Snooker*, by England's great Joe Davis, first published in London in 1949. Davis goes into tremendous detail on such fundamentals as grip, stance, and stroke. In a section called Finding the Angle he dismisses what he calls "one of the most popular tips in the game," that of aiming the cueball at the center of an imaginary ball frozen to the object ball at the point opposite the pocket. I sat up straight when I read these words because I suggested that very thing in *Byrne's Standard Book* for beginners who can't get the hang of cut shots. Davis writes: "It is a very plausible theory, but it happens to be untrue. It might stand you in good stead when the object ball has only a foot or fifteen inches to travel to the pocket; if any more it will let you down. I have tested the theory very thoroughly, placing a ball in the (combination) position, carefully lining the cueball on it, and sending it there with all the care and skill I possess. Further, I have induced others to try. In my experiments I have found that sighting on this principle is always too thick . . . and you can take it that I have made my tests as nearly foolproof as is humanly possible."

He drops the subject soon after and doesn't relate it to the phenomenon of throw with frozen balls, but he gave me the incentive to get to a table and run some tests of my own. I felt I was onto something important. I wanted to see if a cut shot threw as much as a frozen two-ball combination at the same angle, as I suspected, and Davis had given me a simple way of finding out.

The subject here discussed is of vital importance to three-cushion players as well as pool players. A misunderstanding of what direction an object ball will travel after an impact leads to kiss-outs. For pool players, it means balls failing to go into pockets.

Look at Diagram 19, shot number 1. This was my first experiment.

Freeze the 1 and 2 so that the combination line (the line of centers) is directed through the center of the corner pocket. Place the cueball as shown. The 1-ball represents the imaginary ball; that is, where the cueball will be at the moment of contact if the 2 is to be cut to the corner pocket, according to the theory I am trying to debunk. Aim the cueball at the dead center of the 1, use no English, and when you feel your stroke and aim are grooved, ask a friend to remove the 1. Pull the trigger and you will find that the 2 hits the rail around the point marked A. The 2 was thrown by a cueball with no English. Set the combination up again and shoot it as diagrammed without removing the 1-ball. Again the 2 will hit the rail at A. The throw is the same in each case.

Excited, I called the man who serves as my technical consultant in matters like this, Bob Jewett. When I described on the phone what I had

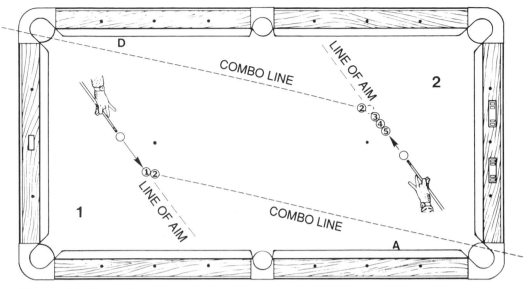

Diagram 19. Throw shots

done, he thought for a moment, then suggested that maybe I had unconsciously influenced the results by altering the hit on the object ball. He said a better test would be to use a three-ball combination, which would remove all doubt.

Back at the table, I set up shot 2 in Diagram 19. You can do it, too. Use the side of a wooden triangle to form a straight line of four frozen balls. Freeze the 2-ball to the end of the line so that it is aimed directly into the corner pocket. Now remove the ball it was frozen to, shown in the diagram by a dashed circle. As you can see, if you drive the cueball into the 5, the 3 pops out of the other end and must occupy the precise space the imaginary ball was in. The 3 must contact precisely the point on the 2 opposite the corner pocket. Shoot and you'll see that the 2 will hit point D.

Using the same experimental setup, I thought of a further confirming experiment. Look at Diagram 20, shot number 3. The 1, 3, 4, and 5 are frozen together in a straight line. The 1 and 2 are aimed at a point on the end rail so that if the cueball is driven into the 5 the 2 will be pocketed. Try the combination a few times to find out where the 2 must be aimed to be made. (The point will vary with the stickiness of the balls.) Once you have found it, set the arrangement up again and carefully remove the 1-ball. Shoot the 5-4-3 combination into the 2 and you will find that it will throw into the pocket just as if the 1 was still there.

Friction between the balls is sufficient to carry the object ball slightly off line as well as to impart a slight spin to it. Throw is insignificant on full hits because the object ball is not given a sideways "rub." It is insignificant on very thin hits because the passing ball is not in contact with the object ball long enough for the friction to act; also the balls are not pressed together

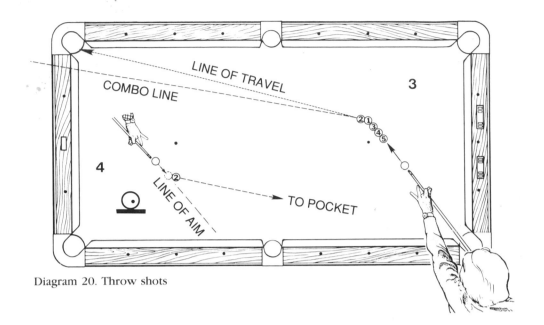

Diagram 20. Throw shots

hard enough for solid contact to be made. This reasoning can be tested.

Set up shot 4 in Diagram 20, which is the same as shot 1. Aim a two-ball frozen combination at the corner pocket. Aim directly through the center of the first ball, and when you are ready to shoot have a friend remove the first ball. This time, though, use right English so that when the cueball hits the 2-ball there will be no "rubbing" action. (The amount of English, of course, to eliminate rubbing entirely depends on speed and the angle of cut; just use judgment.) This time when you pull the trigger you will either make the 2 or come awfully close to it. The outside English has nullified the throw. Now we know why you so often see top players using outside English to "cinch" a shot when position is not critical. (In shot 4, I have placed the cueball quite close to the object ball so that allowing for the curve of the cueball induced by the spin is not an important factor.)

There is a final test. Set up shot 5 as given in Diagram 21. To make the arrangement, first put the cueball on the spot. Set the combination lines so they cross the edges of the pockets to reduce the margin of error. Now back the cueball off three inches. If you shoot between the balls trying to hit them simultaneously, neither one will go because they both will be thrown. The amount of throw will be the same as if you had a third ball on the spot, where the cueball was, and shot into it. Now set the balls up once more. Shoot between them again trying for a simultaneous hit, but this time use side spin. With left English the 1 will go in and the 2 will not. With right English the 2 will go in and the 1 will not.

What further proof is needed that the vast majority of pool players haven't been approaching cut shots correctly?

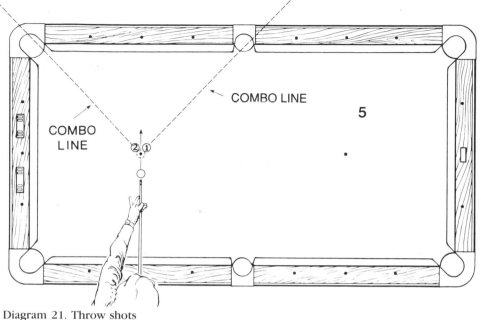

Diagram 21. Throw shots

The Secret of Making Rail Shots

It is surprising how little top players have to know about the physics of the game they play so well. Some carry around notions that are just plain wrong, such as that the cueball on a draw shot goes a short distance through the object ball before backing up (that happens only with a heavy cueball or one that has left the cloth) or that on a follow shot the cueball bounces backward off the object ball before going forward (that happens only when the cueball is lighter than the object ball or when the object ball is supported, as it is on the break shot). Many players use "systems" for certain shots, systems that turn out to be false when analyzed closely. Not too many top players will admit that they play almost entirely by instinct or judgment. One player who would was the late Luther Lassiter. Once when he was in Sacramento, Calif., for a tournament, I asked him if he could find time to give me a few lessons. He replied: "I don't give lessons because I don't know what I'm doing."

I will show you now how to make a shot that is incorrectly described in every instruction book that mentions it. The shot is pocketing a ball that is frozen to the rail. The student is routinely told to hit the ball and the rail at the same time. Such advice may be good enough for beginners, who shouldn't be burdened with too many fine points at the start, but the truth is that when no English or inside English is used the rail must be hit first.

Let's eliminate shots where the frozen ball is only a foot or two from the corner pocket, or where the pockets are easy, or the object ball is encouraged to stay on the rail by a groove in the cloth or by a table that isn't level. The margin of error is so great in those cases that little is proved by experimentation. Consider instead a shot where great accuracy is required, like the upper shot in Diagram 23, which calls for cutting a ball along the rail past the side pocket. If the pockets are tight, the cloth is new, and the table is level, how many times can you make that shot in ten attempts? If you aim to hit the rail and ball at the same time, you will be lucky to make it two or three times in ten. If you hit the rail slightly first, you can quickly learn to make it eight or nine times in ten, as I did.

First, a review of the previous chapter. At the top of Diagram 22, the 1-ball and the 2-ball are frozen and aimed at the pocket at A. If you shoot a cue-ball directly at the center of the 1-ball, as shown, the 2-ball will be thrown forward and will hit the rail near T. That is common knowledge. Now try this: Aim at the precise center of the 1-ball with no English, and just before pulling the trigger ask a friend to remove the 1-ball. If you shoot without changing your aim, the cueball at the moment of contact will occupy the same space as the 1-ball did and the contact point will be exactly opposite the target, just as the instruction books and teachers advise. Yet the 2-ball will hit the rail at T, just as it did when it was part of the combination. If you use outside English (right, in this case) the 2-ball will not throw because the surface of the cueball will not rub against the surface of the 2-ball.

At the bottom of Diagram 22 is a familiar challenge or "bar bet" shot. If the 3-ball combination is struck as shown, the 5-ball will not stay on the rail—it will rebound along the line marked R. The 5-ball will stay on the rail only if the contact point between 4 and 5 is moistened (secretly if you are trying to rob somebody). The point to be made here is that the 4-ball is touching the 5-ball and the rail at the same time, which is exactly where the conventional wisdom suggests the cueball should be if you were simply cutting a single 5-ball up the rail. Yet the 5-ball diverges from the rail. The reason is that it is thrown into the rail and rebounds from it.

Set up the same 3-4-5 combination, but this time don't freeze the 4 and 5. Leave about a one-fourth-inch gap between them. Now hit the 3-ball and the 5 stays on the rail! This demonstration proves the thesis, which is that to run a ball down a rail the rail should be hit first. (In the three-ball combination, the size of the gap depends on how hard you hit it.)

Look again at the cut shot at the top of Diagram 23. To make it consistently, first aim to hit the rail and the ball simultaneously, then change the aim slightly to favor the rail. Don't shoot too hard. No English is needed, but inside English (left, in this case) enables you to hit the rail farther from the object ball than would be the case without English. I'm talking fractions of inches here—hit the rail just *slightly* first.

Why does it work? The explanation is in Diagram 24. Because the object ball throws on simple cut shots, you must slightly overcut them (unless you use outside English). There are two ways that can happen if you hit the rail first. At the left the cueball is shown at the moment of contact with the

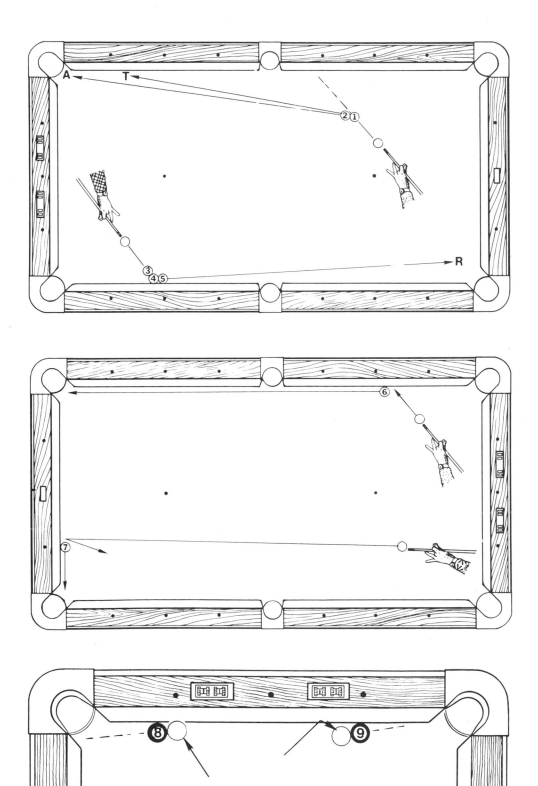

Diagrams 22, 23, and 24: Rail shots

8-ball. The line of centers (dashed line) diverges from the rail, but since the cueball is sinking into the rubber, depressing it more and more, the 8-ball will be thrown into a path parallel to the rail. At the right, the cueball is shown contacting the 9-ball, but after it has depressed the rubber and is rebounding away. This time the line of centers converges with the rail, but since the cueball is leaving the rail the throw effect will act in proper direction and the 9-ball will travel parallel to the rail.

A related shot is the familiar right-angle cut shown at the bottom of Diagram 23. Several books reveal that the secret is to hit the rail first with plenty of English, but none gives the correct reason. When the cueball hits the 7-ball it is emerging from the rubber—the hit is slightly thinner than the geometry it calls for, which is just what you want on a cut shot.

A final note. When the balls are dirty or greasy or covered with chalk, the throw effect is much greater than it is when the balls are clean. The only way to avoid having to guess at how much to allow for throw on cut shots and combinations is to brush the table, wash your hands, and clean the balls before starting play.

When to Cut and When to Throw

It's possible to cut a ball to the left with a level cue and make the cueball go to the left as well, as impossible as it seems. Before explaining how, I want to make sure you understand the underlying geometry and physics.

If you ignore friction between the balls, picking the correct contact point on an object ball is a simple matter: it's the point farthest from the target. Let's say the target is a pocket. Imagine a line from the pocket to the center of the ball and extend it through the ball until it emerges on the other side—that's the contact point. If the cueball hits it, then the object ball will travel along the imagined line to the pocket.

Unfortunately, friction must always be considered, and the effect it will have in throwing the object ball off line can never be calculated precisely. Sticky balls throw more than clean ones. Once a good player is used to the balls, though, he can estimate the amount of friction and throw within a fairly narrow range, often unconsciously.

Ball-to-ball friction complicates the game, but it also increases the player's options when controlling the cueball.

The most basic application of throw on a cut shot is shown at the left of Diagram 25. A beginner might decide that the black ball can't be cut in because of the interfering ball; the point on the black ball farthest from the target is masked by the other ball. A more experienced player knows that

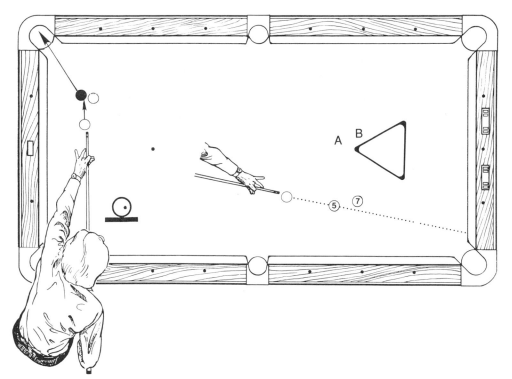

Diagram 25. Throw and cut shots

the ball can be made easily with right spin on the cueball, which throws the object ball to the left.

An advanced application of throw is reducing or increasing the cueball's sideways drift on a cut shot. Consider the shot at the right of Diagram 25. The game is straight pool. The problem is to make the 5-ball and still have an angle on the 7-ball so it can be used to break the pack. It is much better in a case like this to shoot almost straight at the object ball and throw it to the right with left sidespin; if done properly the cueball will move only a little to the left after hitting the object ball.

Or the player may want to maximize the sideways travel of the cueball. In the same position, using right spin on the cueball and a slightly below center hit, the player can overcut the object ball, counting on the sidespin to throw it back on line, and get the cueball to move to the vicinity of A for an angle on a break ball at B.

Now for the solution to the problem posed at the start, cutting a ball to the left and sending the cueball to the left as well.

At the top of Diagram 26, the cueball and the 3-ball are exactly one ball width from the rail. If the balls are only half an inch apart, you may be surprised to know that the 3-ball can be sent along the rail into the corner pocket while at the same time sending the cueball either into the same rail or all the way across the width of the table.

To make the cueball drift to the left, use heavy right English and angle

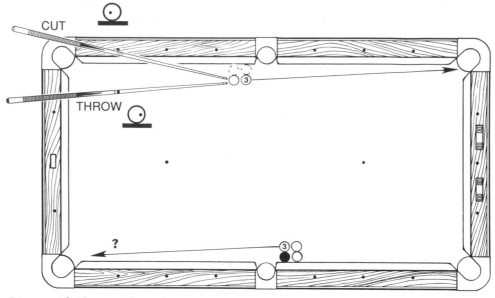

Diagram 26. Throw and cut shots

the cue as if you were cutting the 3-ball *away* from the rail—the English will throw it back to the left and the cueball will go to the left as well. (Something similar, with the cueball frozen to the object ball, is given on page 88 of *Byrne's Standard Book.*) When correctly aimed, the butt of the cue crosses the end rail about six or eight inches from the corner. It is vital to keep the cue as level as possible, for a massé effect would work against you.

To send the cueball all the way across the width of the table, aim the shot as a cut with no English or overcut it with left English.

Many players don't realize that they have so much freedom of cueball action on this shot.

The farther the two balls are apart, the less freedom there is. If the two balls are a full ball width apart, you can still throw the ball into the pocket and make the cueball drift left, but only slightly. When the distance to the first ball is two ball widths, you can stop the cueball dead, but you can't get it to go left. At greater distances, the cueball will drift to the right.

When the distance between the balls is several feet, accuracy becomes a problem. It is still possible to minimize cueball drift by using sidespin, but it becomes harder to make the shot. Many players use *slight* outside English on fairly long cut shots to minimize the throw effect, but to do it effectively they have to be able to allow for squirt (deflection of the cueball off the aiming line toward the side opposite the English) and curve. Each player must determine his own length-of-shot limits depending on his skill, tolerance for risk, and the shot's margin of error.

The position at the bottom of Diagram 26 is given as an item of curiosity, though gamblers might use it as a proposition bet. The cueball and the

3-ball are frozen to balls that are in turn frozen to the rail. The space between them is the width of a cube of chalk. Shooting crisply (no slow rolling), can the 3-ball be made into the corner pocket without moving the black ball? If the black ball even trembles, that counts as "moving," and the shooter loses the bet.

It turns out that if you try to cut the 3-ball in, the black ball will at least quiver. If you shoot straight at the 3 and throw it to the left with right English, the black ball is untouched. The balls compress enough so that the 3-ball is clear of the black ball before it is thrown.

Twenty Keys to a Killer Break

Want to be a consistent winner at eight ball and nine ball? Then you've got to have a crushing break. Players who can splatter the balls all over the table without losing control of the cueball have a big advantage; very often they can run out the game without giving their opponents a chance.

You don't have to be a big brute to break the balls effectively. More important than bulging muscles is proper technique. After watching top pros in action for years, studying videotapes, and interviewing players known for their explosive breaks, I've developed a list of tips. If your break doesn't improve after putting these ideas in action, maybe you should try darts, where accuracy is all and power doesn't count.

1. **Form a looped bridge.** An open or "V" bridge is okay for most pool shots, but when you intend to thrust the cue forward with maximum speed, you'd better circle the cue with your forefinger—it's the only way to make sure the cue will stay on line.

2. **Lengthen your bridge.** Plant your bridge hand on the table a couple of inches farther away from the cueball than you would for a soft shot, say eight or ten inches instead of six or eight. You need extra room for a longer backswing.

3. **Change your grip.** Move your grip hand three or four inches closer to the back end of the cue and grip it firmly to make sure it won't slip. Some players feel that a tight grip using all four fingers adds part of the weight of your arm to the weight of the cue, but the point is arguable.

4. **Forget your wrist.** Whether or not your wrist is locked or loose is unimportant.

5. **Adjust your stance.** If you usually shoot with your chin within a few inches from the cue (which is best for accuracy), stand up a little straighter on the break shot.

6. **Control your stroke.** Take a few vigorous warm-up strokes to prepare yourself for unleashing maximum power and to refine your aim. The

final back swing should be long and slow, like drawing an arrow back in a bow.

7. **Time it.** A good break depends in part on proper timing. The cue should reach its greatest speed at the moment of contact with the cueball. Easier said than done.

8. **Explode.** When you decide to pull the trigger, think of a bomb going off. Try to explode the cue into the cueball.

9. **Follow *straight* through.** The cue tip should hit the cloth a foot or two in front of the cueball. If you consistently follow straight through, then you will consistently send the cue into the cueball accurately.

10. **Freeze.** Lunging on the break adds little or nothing to the speed of the cueball and interferes with accuracy. Better to keep your body still and your head down.

11. **Use the right cue.** A heavy cue isn't necessarily better for breaking because it's harder to control and can't be brought forward as fast as a lighter cue. A powerfully built man can perhaps get more cueball speed with a cue weighing 22 or 23 ounces, but 20 or 21 is the limit for most players. Many pros are now breaking with cues as light as 18 ounces, an ounce or two *lighter* than their regular cues.

12. **Don't elevate.** Keep the cue as level as possible; otherwise the cueball will jump too far off the cloth. Because the butt of the cue is bound to be elevated slightly on the break shot, a really powerful stroke will force the cueball to jump. A jumping cueball is hard to control and often lands on the floor.

13. **Use a hard tip.** The harder the tip the better on the break, for the same reason that hammers are made of steel rather than rubber: the energy absorbed at impact is immediately returned.

14. **Use a stiff cue.** All cues vibrate when struck, but stiff cues vibrate less than flexible or spindly ones. With less energy lost to vibration, more is left to transfer to the cueball.

15. **Avoid sidespin.** Make sure the cue tip hits the cueball exactly in the center or a little below. Sidespin makes the cueball deflect from the aiming line, which makes a direct hit on the pack impossible. Concentrate hard on avoiding sidespin.

16. **Kill the cueball.** Ideally, the cueball should move only a foot or two after hitting the pack. When that happens, almost all of its energy has been imparted to the balls. Strive mightily for a dead-square hit on the apex ball.

17. **Don't scratch.** Scratching is the worst thing that can happen on the break. Avoid it by getting as square a hit as possible on the pack. Don't let the cueball run around the table looking for a pocket.

18. **Relocate the cueball.** Many pros are now breaking from the side of the table rather than the center. The theory is that there is less chance

of scratching in one of the side pockets, there is more chance of making the apex ball in the side, and there is a better chance, in nine ball, of getting the 9 moving.

19. **Practice.** Few players practice the break shot, maybe because they don't like to rack balls. A shot so important, though, deserves to be worked on. Even a small improvement will pay big dividends.

20. **Keep smiling.** Nobody's perfect, so don't let failure get you down. The best players in the world make a ball on the break in nine ball only three times in five, and they make the 9-ball only one time in 35.

Of all the elements that go into a good break shot, one towers over the others in importance: an accurate hit on the pack. Try above all else to hit the apex ball as squarely as possible. Even if you are so delicate and petite that your break shot wouldn't break an egg, the balls will spread well if hit squarely.

Searching for the Perfect Break Cue

The opening break is by far the most important shot in eight ball and nine ball, yet there is no general agreement on how it should be done. Should the cueball be placed in the center, a few inches from the center, two feet from the center, or so close to the side that you must bridge from the rail? At major tournaments you can find all of the above. You can also find a variety of grips, strokes, and stances.

Over the last couple of years, the cueball position on the break has been migrating toward the side of the table in nine-ball tournaments. Breaking from the side, players claim, tends to cut the chance of scratching, seems to get the 9-ball moving more, and increases the chances of pocketing the 1-ball. No studies have been done to support the claims.

Even the question of what cue to use on the break has never been settled. Should it be long, short, thin, fat, light, or heavy? Should you even use a different cue on the break? Nick Varner (who weighs only 115 pounds and yet has a powerful break) breaks with the same 19-ounce cue he plays with on the grounds that he doesn't want something unfamiliar in his hands for such a crucial shot. The disadvantage, he admits, is that his tip flattens and wears out too fast.

Not too long ago, most players thought that a heavy cue was best for the break; now the consensus is swinging in the opposite direction. Mike Sigel, to cite a conspicuous example, plays with a 20 and breaks with an 18.

What weight is best for the break? The goal is the greatest possible speed on the cueball and the squarest possible hit on the pack; the problem is that the harder you hit the cueball the less control you have over it.

I once tried to solve part of the problem with the help of field research and the laws of nature. Forgetting accuracy, what weight cue gives the maximum cueball speed? That was the question put to science. A cue weighing 1 ounce would crumple against the cueball; a cue weighing 100 pounds couldn't be brought forward fast enough. Somewhere in between was the ideal weight, and a band of courageous researchers tried to find it.

Experiments that were comical if not conclusive were conducted in my garage and driveway on April 18, 1989. While no members of the Nobel Prize committee were present, there was no shortage of frightening heavyweights. Assisting with cues of various weights, clipboards, calculators, and tape measures were Mike Shamos, who is a member of the physics faculty at Carnegie-Mellon in Pittsburgh; Bob Jewett, who is a research scientist for Hewlett-Packard; Tony Annigoni, who once beat Jim Rempe to win a nine-ball tournament in Sacramento, Calif.; and Lee Simon, who owns a store called Billiards Unlimited and is an expert on cues and tables. Several neighbors and passersby refused to identify themselves and threatened to call the police.

Here was the situation: Simon was setting up a pool table (a black-and-brass Gandy) in my garage. Before the rails were attached there was an opportunity to try an experiment suggested by Robert Callahan, a science professor at Morehead State University in Kentucky. In the absence of electronic equipment, a cueball's speed can be calculated by shooting it off the end of the table and measuring how far it flies before hitting the floor . . . or, in my case, the driveway.

I remembered most of the applicable ballistics equations from engineering school, but to make sure I had them right I consulted with Dr. George Onoda of IBM's Watson Research Center in Yorktown Heights, N.Y. It was Onoda who studied videotapes and oscilloscopes to calculate that the cueball averages about 24 mph when top pros break in nine ball. His results appeared in the April 1989 *Billiards Digest*.

The main equation for the Callahan test is simple: $S = 1.76D$ (approximately), where S is the speed of the cueball in miles per hour and D is the horizontal distance in feet measured from the end of the table to the spot the cueball hits the ground. This assumes that the table is 29 inches high. A cueball traveling 24 mph when it leaves the end of the table will land 13.5 feet away.

After the driveway was covered with blankets, we took turns shooting the cueball off the table as hard as we could, using six cues ranging in weight from 9.5 ounces to 25.9 ounces. Sixty-seven shots were taken and measured. Jewett recorded the results and later plotted them on graph paper. No cueballs were lost and no windows were broken. An average of 1.374 cans of beer was consumed per researcher.

The results were suggestive but not conclusive, partly because of the inconsistency of the shooters (distances varied as much as 20 percent from shot to shot) and because we didn't have a cue for each step of the way in the sensitive range, which is from about 18 to 21 ounces.

Simon had the three best shots, reaching 23.72 mph with a 20-ounce cue, 23.29 mph with a 19.5 ouncer, and a surprising 22.85 mph with a 17.9 ouncer. Nobody topped 20 mph with the 25.9-ounce graphite "break" cue.

Two cueballs were used, a pool ball weighing 5.9 ounces and an ivory billiard ball weighing 7.35 ounces. The sixth and seventh greatest speeds (22.42 mph and 22.28 mph) were achieved by Simon using the 19.5-ounce cue and hitting the 7.35-ounce ball, which argues strongly in favor of the trend toward lighter break cues. The trials also argued against using a very heavy cue.

When Professor Callahan ran the same sort of test in Kentucky, he managed, in one glorious case when everything went right, to give the cueball a speed of 30 mph with a 20-ounce cue even though he weighs only 145 pounds. How did he do it? By practicing karate for 15 years. Throwing his body forward and twisting his torso so that everything reached top speed at the moment of impact added considerably to the speed of his cue. Accuracy, though, went out the window.

If you could bring a heavy cue forward as fast as a light one, you could break harder because the speed of the cueball depends both on the weight and speed of the cue. The formula is not complicated. To find out how fast the cueball will go after being hit by a cue, double the weight of the cue, multiply it by the speed of the cue, and divide the result by the sum of the weight of the cue and the ball.

As an example, say the cue weighs three times the ball (18 ounces to 6 ounces). In that case, the cueball will leave the tip at a speed 1.5 times the speed of the cue. If the cue weighs four times the ball (24 to 6), then the cueball will be given a speed 1.6 times the speed of the cue.

In other words, by adding 33 percent to the weight of the cue you are chasing only a 6.6 percent gain in cueball speed. And because you can't swing a heavy cue as fast, the potential gain is even less. When you also consider the importance of precision and control, which are easier to achieve with a light cue, then it seems to me there is no longer any argument. Light cues are best. Mike Sigel is right.

There is corroboration in the 1984 book *Sports Science*, by Peter J. Brancazio, professor of physics at Brooklyn College. While he doesn't discuss the break shot in pool, he minutely examines something similar, the collisions between baseballs and bats. On the subject of transfer of energy, he writes on page 230: ". . . it is more effective for the batter to put his effort into swinging a lighter bat at higher speed—or, in other words, that bat speed is a more important consideration than weight." And a light baseball bat, like a light cue, can be swung more accurately than a heavy one.

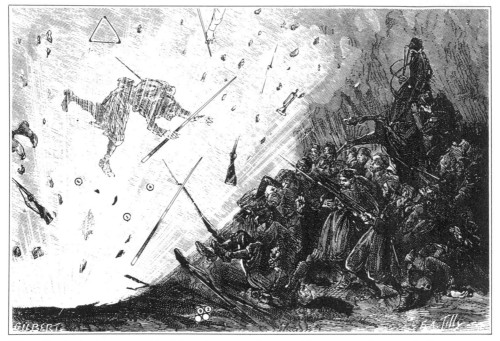

When the tests were over, the laboratory was destroyed by a mysterious explosion.

What weight bat or cue is best for you, of course, depends on the size of your wingspan, the strength of your arms, and whether or not you have a black belt in karate.

Want to do some research of your own? Then do what I'm going to do next time: Use a radar gun.

Note: In addition to the gentlemen named above, I wish to thank Pat Fleming and David Howard for educational discussions on the break shot.

The Truth about Bank Shots

More baloney has been written about bank shots in pool than almost anything else in life. Most books that discuss the subject state or assume that the angle of incidence equals the angle of reflection, which is true if you are dealing with light rays bouncing off mirrors but not pool balls bouncing off cushions.

The point is easily proven on a billiard table. Freeze the ball in a corner and shoot it without English in the midpoint of the opposite long rail. It will not bank into the other corner as the equal-angle predicts. It will go "long" and will hit the short rail at least a half-diamond from the corner. The reason is the natural roll on the ball, which causes its path to bend forward after leaving the first rail. If you hit the ball hard enough so that it slides rather than rolls into the rail, the rebound angle more closely matches the angle of approach.

The same thing is true on a pool table when you try to bank an object ball. If you hit it so hard that the object ball doesn't have time to begin rolling naturally before it hits the rail, it will come short. That bank shots are shortened by increased speed is widely known, but the reason has never before appeared in print.

Also rarely, if ever, written about is the tremendous effect English has on bank shots. The English can be imparted to the object ball either by cutting it or by spinning the cueball. An understanding of the principle will greatly shorten the time it will take you to become a good banker.

As you now know, on simple cut shots the object ball gets "thrown" just like a two-ball frozen combination—unless outside English is used, which eliminates the friction when the cueball hits the object ball. In other words, when using center ball or inside English on a cut shot, you must slightly overcut the ball. The same factor must be considered on bank shots along with an additional crucial variable: transferred English.

Because of speed, spin, and throw, the various geometric and mirror-image banking systems aren't worth much.

Consider the top position in Diagram 27, which is familiar to most players because it is the starting point in many trick shots. Struck as shown, the striped ball will go into corner pocket Y and the black ball will bank into side pocket Z. In setting it up, the two frozen balls must be directed straight across the table as indicated by the dashed line; the reason is that the striped ball in rubbing across the face of the black ball will throw it slightly to the right and will also give it a little right English. Unfortunately, most players who know how to set up the trick shot don't apply the principle to shots that come up in their games.

At the bottom of the diagram, the goal is to bank the black ball into

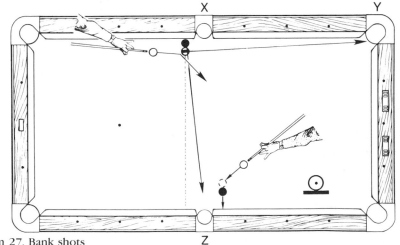

Diagram 27. Bank shots

side pocket X. The dashed ball shows where the cueball will be if it contacts the object ball directly opposite the cushion. In theory, that should drive the object ball straight into the rail as indicated (provided there is no English on the cueball). In practice, however, the black ball gets thrown forward and hits the rail a little closer to the side pocket than the arrow suggests, and in addition is given a slight sidespin by the passing cueball. The result is that it banks in the side. Most good players make such easy banks consistently on instinct and experience, not because they have a clear understanding of what happens.

In Diagram 28 the object is to bank the black ball into the side pocket from three different cueball positions. If a center ball hit is used on the cueball, it may surprise you to know that a different contact point is required on the rail for each of the three starting points. While experimenting with

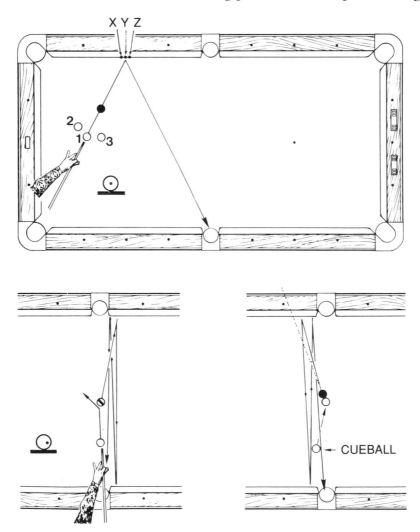

Diagrams 28 and 29: Bank shots

this, mark the cueball and object ball positions on the cloth with chalk so the balls can quickly and accurately be respotted.

After marking the object ball location, find position 1 for the cueball so that a straight-ahead hit at soft speed will result in a successful bank. Have a friend mark the contact point on the rail (shown here as Y). Now mark cueball positions 2 and 3, roughly six inches on either side of position 1. You will find that to bank the black ball from position 2 you will have to drive it into the rail a little to the left of Y, at a point I have marked X, because the black ball will pick up a little running English from the cueball. From starting point 3 the contact point on the rail is on the other side of Y, at the point marked Z, because a small amount of reverse (holdup) English is on the object ball. These statements hold true only if you use no English. With "running" English (right from position 2 and left from position 3), friction at the instant of contact can be eliminated, along with throw and transfer English, and point Y becomes correct.

Further understanding of banks can be gained by trying the shot from position 1 with English on the cueball. With heavy right English, you must drive the object ball into point Z. With heavy left English you must hit point X. With lesser amounts of English, of course, the effect is reduced.

The two shots in Diagram 29, which could come up in any game, illustrate the points in an entertaining way. Both are in *Byrne's Treasury of Trick Shots*. In the shot at the left, the striped ball is in the exact center of the table. Nevertheless, it can be triple-banked in the side by using extreme right English on the cueball.

At the right in Diagram 29 is a surprising shot that makes intermediate players gasp. The black ball is on the center spot and the white ball is frozen against it so that the two are lined up as indicated by the dashed line. Strike the white ball full and the black ball can be made to triple bank in the side in a beautiful demonstration of throw and transfer English.

Students serious about mastering bank shots should also take a look at the holdup double bank on page 146 of my trick shot book and at the three examples on page 99 of *Byrne's Standard Book*.

Facts about Follow, Skidding, and Banks

In my videotape on how to play pool, I state categorically that when you want the cueball to follow the object ball, it is useless to hit the cueball higher than 70 percent of its diameter, but I don't take the time to explain why. I'll take the time now, for the point is important.

In his great book on the physics of billiards, published early in the last century, Gustave Coriolus showed that when the cueball is struck 70 percent of its diameter above the bottom (a hair less than halfway from the center to the top), it starts out immediately with natural roll; that is, the ball and the cloth are in solid contact without sliding of any kind. The question is, will a higher hit give the cueball extra topspin? Yes, but it is almost impossible to demonstrate it under game conditions.

My technical adviser, Bob Jewett of Hewlett-Packard, came up with a simple test to get to the bottom of the matter. The results amazed me.

Place an object ball in the center of the table, as in Diagram 30, and the cueball near the head rail, at point R. Hit the cueball in the center (no topspin), and bank the object ball to point P, or thereabouts. At that speed, the cueball will be rolling naturally by the time it reaches the object ball, and the natural forward roll will cause it to follow to roughly point F. On the table I used for the test, the cueball rolls about a third as far as the object ball. Mark on the table, or write down, or remember where the two balls come to rest.

Return the object ball to the center of the table and put the cueball an inch or two away from it, on the point marked T. Bank the object ball the same distance, but this time put as much topspin on the cueball as you can. Will the cueball follow farther than it did when it was only rolling naturally? The surprising answer is no! Provided the two shots are hit with the same speed (as shown by the distance the object ball is driven), the follow on the cueball is the same. You might occasionally be able to put *slightly* more follow on the cueball with high topspin, but the difference in the length of the follow will be too slight to matter in practical terms.

Think of the money you could make with this information if you were unscrupulous! Bet a top player that you can put just as much follow on the cueball by hitting the center as he can by hitting it high, and watch him

Diagram 30. Follow, skidding, and banks

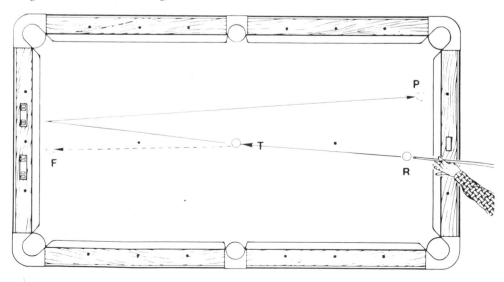

reach for his wallet! Just make sure you start with the cueball far enough away from the object ball so that it has time to begin rolling naturally before contact. Your hapless dupe can put the cueball anywhere he wants and can hit the cueball as high as he wants and he won't be able to make the cueball follow any farther than you did. (Either throw out shots where the object ball doesn't bank to the right place or keep track of every shot by dividing the length of the drive by the length of the follow. The ratio will remain close to constant.)

The practical implications of this experiment are (1), that hitting the cueball more than halfway between the center and the edge on a follow shot (and perhaps on draw and sidespin shots as well) is useless and merely increases the chance of a miscue and (2), that if the cueball is rolling naturally or has been struck halfway from the center to the top, the length of the follow depends only on how hard the cueball is hit.

At another point in the videotape I state flatly that the various systems for calculating bank shots don't work well because they are based on the assumption that the angle of the approach to the rail equals the angle of departure. Again, I don't take the time to fully explain why.

Follow, or topspin, or natural forward roll are the culprits that make banking a guessing game rather than a geometry problem. If a ball has forward roll on it, it will bend "forward" on leaving the rail, thus making the apparent angle of departure less than the angle of approach.

The effect of topspin off the rail is demonstrated dramatically in the billiard trick shot I call Bulldog Brink Bends the Ball (page 273 in *Byrne's Treasury of Trick Shots*). The same idea can be applied to pool. In Diagram 31, it looks impossible to bank the cueball and make the ball near the diagonally opposite pocket because of the interfering balls. However! Hit

Diagram 31. Follow, skidding, and banks

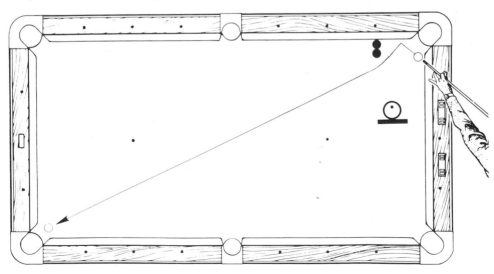

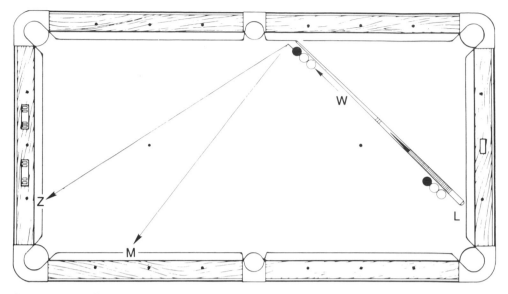

Diagram 32. Follow, skidding, and banks

the cueball three-fourths of the way up, giving it natural forward roll, and it will bend around the blocking balls. Don't shoot hard.

To show the tremendous influence slide and follow have on bank shots, Bob Jewett suggested an idea that I have used in Diagram 32. Set up two three-ball combinations along the same line (put a cue on the table and use it as a guide in aligning the balls), one close to the rail, one four feet away. Put the cueball at W, hit the upper combination with medium speed, and watch where the black ball banks. It will hit the opposite rail at about point M.

Now remove those three balls, place the cueball at L, and hit the second combination at the same speed. This time the black ball (the front ball) will bank to the other side of the corner pocket, at point Z! The reason for the tremendous difference in the angle is that in the first case the banked ball was sliding into the rail, while in the second case the banked ball had time to acquire a natural forward roll. This demonstration would make another good bar bet, for few players, even the best ones, would be able to predict the results with much accuracy.

And now the solution to another mystery, why an object ball sometimes "skids." Once every 100 shots or so, when you are trying a cut shot, the cueball seems to "grab" the object ball and throw it forward. The object ball slides after the hit instead of rolling, and sometimes even hops a little. Irving Crane has said that when this happens the object ball acts like a sliding ashtray instead of a ball.

I've written before about the weird effects that are possible if you chalk the contact points between balls (pages 152–153 in my trick shot book). Chalk greatly increases the friction between the balls, making them behave for an instant like cog wheels. If you chalk your cue and strike a cueball, you implant a nice big chalk mark on it, and if by chance that chalk mark is oriented in such a way that it strikes the object ball at the moment of contact, skid occurs. On a cut shot, the object ball gets thrown forward; on a straight-in shot, if the cueball is rolling, the chalk spot strikes the object ball a downward blow, making it hop and slide.

Steve Davis, the world's best snooker player, lost the world title in 1985 when he blew an easy cut on the final 7-ball. Skid was probably the reason. As ridiculous as it sounds, Davis, and you, too, if you are ever faced with a cut shot for all the money, would have been better off *removing* all chalk from his tip. Attention, hustlers! Spitting on your opponent's tip might cost you the game!

The Importance of the Half-ball Hit

Very few players have clear in their minds three important facts: 1) To make a naturally rolling cueball deflect at a given angle off an object ball, there are almost always two places the object ball can be struck; 2) In terms of the angle the cueball is deflected when hitting an object ball, the half-ball hit is most resistant to error; 3) The half-ball hit causes the naturally rolling cueball to deflect the maximum amount.

Diagram 33 illustrates what is meant by the term *half-ball hit*. Note that the center of the cueball is directed at the edge of the object ball. It's a useful concept in three cushion because it provides the shooter with something specific to aim at in many situations. The player familiar with the deflection angle in a half-ball hit can often eliminate one variable (the amount of object ball to hit) and concentrate on speed and spin. The great Jay Bozeman once told me that when he was jousting for the world three-cushion crown with Willie Hoppe and Welker Cochran in the 1930s and 40s he went for the half-ball hit whenever possible.

The importance of the half-ball hit derives from its resistance to error.

Diagram 33. The half-ball hit

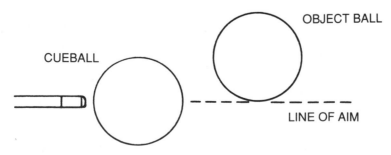

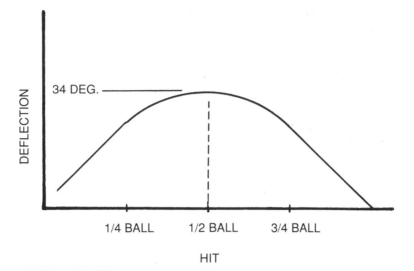

Diagram 34. The half-ball hit

That is, you can hit the object ball slightly fuller or slightly thinner than half and the deflection of the cueball's path will still be about the same. For the balls and cloth used today, the deflection angle, for practical purposes, is 34 degrees.

The resistance-to-error effect can be seen in the simple graph in Diagram 34. The curve represents the amount of deflection of the cueball's path for various hits. At the left end the curve is at zero because the cueball's path hardly changes at all for a very fine grazing hit. The curve climbs as you move along the horizontal scale because the thicker the object ball is hit the more the cueball is deflected. The maximum, 34 degrees, is reached when the hit is half a ball. From there, for fuller hits, the curve declines because the cueball *follows through* the object ball. The curve reaches zero again at the right end, which represents a full-in-the-face hit, when the cueball follows straight through the object ball without going right or left.

Two practical conclusions can be drawn from the graph. One is the resistance to error of the half-ball hit. Note that the half-ball hit occurs at the flat part of the curve—a little to the right or left doesn't make much difference in the height of the curve or, in other words, in the amount of the deflection. The second point is that to get a given rebound angle off the ball, the ball can be hit in two different places. The cueball is deflected the same amount for a one-quarter-ball hit as for a three-quarter-ball hit (about 27.5 degrees in practice). This last point is made use of frequently by three-cushion players trying to miss a kiss or play position—they estimate the path the cueball must take from the first object ball to the first rail, then they decide whether to drive the cueball ahead or cut it to one side. In either case they hit the same point on the first rail.

Caution—I'm talking only about naturally rolling cueballs. Sliding, top-spinning, or backspinning cueballs give very different results.

Speed, interestingly, has no effect on the deflection angle if it is properly measured, but for the examples in this discussion I'm considering moderate to soft. That speed has no effect is a point made by George Onoda, a scientist at IBM's Watson Research Center in Yorktown Heights, N.Y. It is true that the harder the cueball strikes the object ball the farther it will travel along the right-angle line before bending forward (the parabolic curve is flatter), but after the topspin is spent and the cueball is once again traveling in a straight line, that line, if projected backward, will always form an angle of 34 degrees with the original aiming line. For a full explanation, see Dr. Onoda's article in *The American Journal of Physics,* May 1989.

Now for a valuable practical application, the so-called in-off spot shot. In Diagram 35 the 1-ball is on the foot spot, the pay ball is hanging on the lip, and you have the cueball in hand behind the headstring. Should you cut the 1-ball into the 9-ball or go for the billiard shot? The billard shot is far better, provided you put the cueball in the right place to start with. That place is two inches to the right of the head spot. From there you simply go for the half-ball hit on the 1-ball. The cueball will carom toward the center of the corner pocket with wonderful accuracy. Try it ten times each way and you'll be convinced.

Two more applications of the half-ball spot shot are given in Diagram 36. Suppose the 9-ball is at point a, and the 8-ball is on the spot at g. The object is to pocket the 9 with a carom off the 8. You know that a half-ball hit with the cueball at point d will cause the cueball to cross point b. To make the cueball cross a instead and thus cut the 9 into the corner, place the cueball at point e. Since the distance from d to g is roughly 50 percent

Diagram 35. The half-ball hit

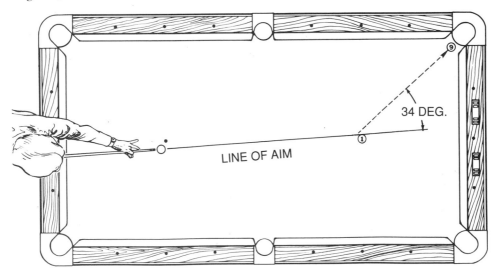

LINE OF AIM

34 DEG.

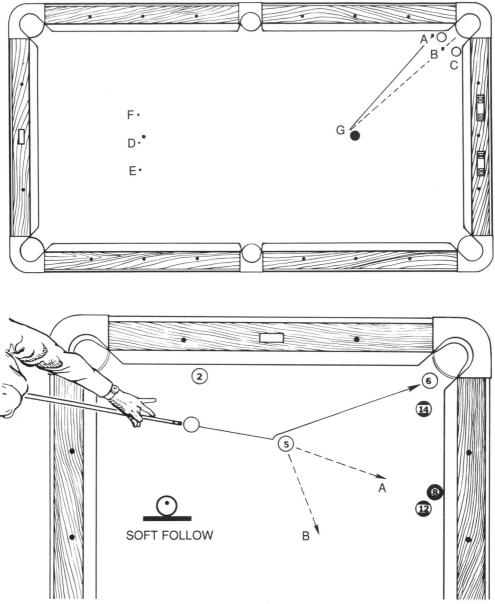

Diagrams 36 and 37: The half-ball hit

more than from g to b, it is necessary to make the distance from d to e 50 percent more than from b to a.

If the 9-ball is at point c, then use a half-ball hit off the 8-ball starting from point f.

To drive home the idea that the object ball can be struck in two places for a given angle of cueball deflection, I present Diagram 37, a position from a game of eight ball. The 2, 5, and 6 are open, but the 8 is trapped.

What should be done? Some might try to cut the 6 in with draw, hoping to knock the 14 into the 8, but that is not too promising in the given situation.

Without knocking the 8 loose, though, there is no way to run out. Consider the carom off the 5. Most pool players who wanted to make the 6 by caroming the cueball off the 5 would consider only the thin hit, driving the 5 along line B. Better here is the full hit, sending the 5 along line A and into the cluster. The cueball follows through the 5 into the 6. After the 6 the 2 is waiting, then the 5 and 8 (with a little luck). There is no need to hit this shot hard. Just use plenty of high follow and enough speed to barely make the 6 without scratching.

The Magic of Massé—Explained

Very few things in life turn people on more than a well-executed massé shot. A cueball that seems to defy the laws of physics by making a right-angle turn and gaining speed is an exhilarating sight for spectators. For the players, making one of the big, sweeping massé shots during competition is a thrill beyond compare. Joy reigns no matter how bad you are getting beat or how much money you are losing.

Certain geometrical secrets of the shot haven't been discussed in print since 1835. That was the year Gaspard Gustave Coriolis published his great work on the mathematics of colliding spheres, namely, *Theorie Mathematique des Effects du Jeu de Billard*. The book, which has never been translated into English, is unsurpassed on the physics of billiards.

Ponder Diagram 38, which is a view of the cueball from above. Assume that the cue is elevated to an angle of 70 or 80 degrees (not quite vertical)

Diagram 38. Massé shots

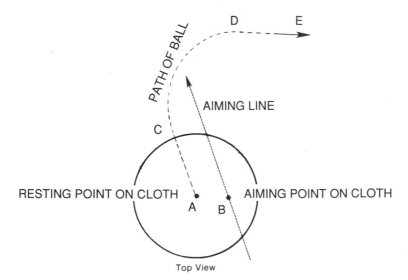

and that it will strike the cueball on the right side and a little behind center. Point A is the spot on the cloth on which the cueball rests. Point B is the point on the cloth the tip would hit if you followed straight through. In other words, point B is the spot on the cloth you aim at during a massé shot.

Point B must be chosen with care, unless you are so experienced that you can trust judgment alone—as practically all top players do when attempting massé shots. In the diagram, note how the cueball starts out in a direction parallel to the aiming line, then bends to the right. At point D the curve ends and the ball continues in a straight line to and beyond point E. The delicious secret is that line DE is parallel to AB. Thus you can make the cueball take the desired final direction by properly locating point B. This very helpful fact will come as news to practically every player in the United States and takes much of the guesswork out of what until this moment has been one of the game's most mysterious shots.

In planning the shot, you first choose the line of aim, AC, then how far you want the ball to travel before the curve begins, and finally the direction you want it to take after the curve is over. The lengths of AC and CD depend on the amount of elevation of the cue, how far off center you hit the cueball, how much force you use, and the friction between the tip and the ball and the ball and the cloth. Such variables require touch and judgment, but at least one essential factor can be calculated rather precisely, and that is the final direction. Once you have decided what you want the final direction of the ball, DE, to be, simply pick a point B so that AB is parallel to DE. When addressing the cueball, imagine the point where it touches the cloth. Imagine a point B on the cloth that will produce the desired final direction and aim your cue through the cueball at point B.

Naturally, your tip must be properly dressed and chalked to have much chance of success.

Before continuing, a couple of basic points. A massé shot is a kind of miscue. The cueball gets squeezed between the tip and the cloth in the same way a watermelon seed can be shot from between thumb and forefinger. You also hit down on the cueball when you want it to jump; it doesn't jump in a massé shot because the cueball is smothered by the tip.

Hold the cue against your cheek so that it crosses your ear. If you can't form a bridge on the table, or if you have to hit the ball hard, use a freehand bridge with the forearm pressed against the body for as much solidity as possible. Willie Hoppe's *Billiards As It Should Be Played* has several good photos of the correct stance and grip. Sometimes you can lift a knee onto the rail and base your bridge on that.

Not much force is required unless you want the cueball to go several feet before curving. In the small massés typical of straight billiards, where the total travel is only a few inches, the force is hardly more than dropping the cue onto the ball. The results can be magical.

Students often ask how far off center they should hit the cueball. The answer depends on the shot, your tip, and your stroke.

In Diagram 39, assume that the player, intending to put draw on the cueball, is hitting the ball as low as he can without danger of miscuing. That is, the perpendicular from point G, the center of mass of the cueball, and H on the aiming line, is as long as it can be. Each player should know how long GH can be on a standard draw shot. The rule is this: GH is the same no matter how much the cue is elevated. That is, when the cue is elevated, hit the cueball no farther off center than you would on a deep draw shot.

Now for the line of aim. Diagram 40 shows a position that might come up in nine ball. If you know what you are doing, it is not too difficult to skim the 8 and make the cueball curve into the 9 for a winner. Establish the aiming line with a level cue as shown—in this example you want a thin hit on the 8. Now imagine a vertical plane of glass intersecting the table and entirely containing your cue and the line of aim. Lift the cue to the elevated position (between 70 and 80 degrees from the horizontal), always keeping it within the imaginary plane of glass, and pick an aiming point on the cloth as explained above. A soft stroke is required to make the cueball path curve quickly and to avoid following the 9-ball in (Diagram 41).

In every several hundred points in the game of three-cushion billiards, opportunities arise for massé shots. Perhaps the easiest possible position is given in Diagram 42, left. Straight backspin is all that is required, but you need a steeply elevated cue to make the cueball hit the first rail twice. If you can't make it in ten tries, forget your dreams of making a living as an exhibition player. (For the geometrically inclined, on this shot both point A and B are on the aiming line. Refer to Diagram 38.)

Diagram 39. Massé shots

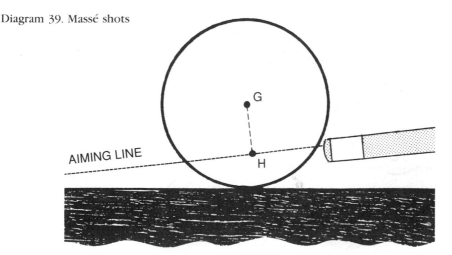

AIMING LINE

G

H

SIDE VIEW

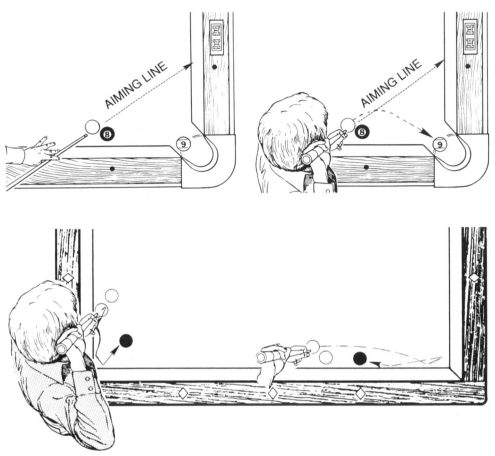

Diagrams 40, 41, and 42: Massé shots

At the right in Diagram 42 is a shot I saw Raymond Ceulemans try in Europe. The great Belgian champion, who has a very secure massé stroke (everything about his game is secure), went lightly off the white, curved around the red, and doubled the rail in the corner. It was an ideal that would have occurred only to a player used to games like straight billiards and balkline, which call for mastery of massé.

When and How to Shoot Jump Shots

Some old-timers claim that 50 years ago anybody who tried a jump shot in a money game would have gotten a fistfight for his trouble, yet the technique has long been legal in the United States in both pool and billiards. At one time, in fact, jumping even the cueball all the way off the table was not considered a foul in billiards provided the point was scored. Quoting from a 1925 rule book published by Brunswick-Balke-Collender: "Jump shots are legitimate in all carom games. If an object ball or cueball be forced off the table, there is no penalty when a counting stroke is made, the count stands, the cueball is placed on the head spot, and the striker continues his inning."

In three-cushion billiards, there is no way to send the cueball off the table after scoring a point, and in that game a player's inning is over when the cueball hits the floor. Under old American professional rules for three cushion, however, it was O.K. to send the first object ball off the table—to miss a kiss, for example, or accidentally—but such dangerous flamboyance is not permitted under the rules that now govern international play.

In snooker, jumps of all kinds are barred. When I was in England in 1984, I questioned several officials on the point. The cueball must not leave the cloth, period. You can't even make it jump a little to get by an edge of an interfering ball. To do so is a foul. That is a poor rule, for great things are possible when players are allowed to play the game in three dimensions.

In the last ten years or so in the United States, the jump shot has . . . well, it has reached new heights. A dramatic example of what is possible can be demonstrated by Mike Massey. With a cueball at one end of the table and an object ball eight feet away, he can jump entirely over an interfering ball, pocket the object ball, and *draw* the cueball back the length of the table. My mouth fell open when I first saw him do it, and my jaw still aches. Such feats are beyond normal people, but many jump shots are not particularly difficult.

Look at the shot in Diagram 43. The game is eight ball. You have an easy cut shot on the last spot, but how can you get past the two stripes to get position on the 8? If you elevate the cue about 45 degrees, it is not hard to jump over the interfering balls and get the cueball to the other end of

Diagram 43. Jump shots

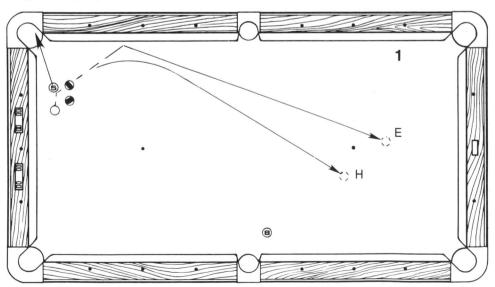

the table . . . to the position marked E, for example. If other balls block that solution, you can try a jump draw, elevating the cue as before but applying backspin. When the cueball lands beyond the interfering balls, its path will bend in the way shown by the line terminating at H.

George Conner of Fort Wayne, Ind., is especially fond of jump draw shots and I'm grateful to him for calling my attention to some of the uses for them.

Shot 2 in Diagram 44 is a little-known application of the jump shot. The problem is to make the 8-ball, which is not quite straight in, and get the cueball down the table. It might be possible to do it with a powerful

Diagrams 44 and 45: Jump shots

follow shot, but what if interfering balls make that impossible? Use a jump shot. If you can make the cueball jump several inches in the air and land on the nose of the cushion, not as hard as it sounds, it will scoot down the table as desired, sometimes all the way to the other end.

Shot 3 is an amazing Great Escape. Believe it or not, it is possible to make the 2-ball in the corner without scratching in the side. The trick is make the cueball jump just enough to hit the upper back rim of the pocket so that it bounces back on the table, avoiding both the hole and the floor. Whether or not the cueball will come to rest at R is, of course, not for me to say. The odds of accomplishing this in a game are slim to none, but it makes a good challenge bet. Some side pockets are friendlier to this shot than others. The shot was shown to me by Ricky Wright. If the angle into the first ball isn't too steep, it is also possible to avoid the scratch by using a soft massé, as suggested to me by Jeff Olney, a sailor based in Hawaii.

In shot 4, Diagram 45, which is straighter than shot 3, the challenge is not only to avoid scratching but to get the cueball in position for a decent shot at the 9-ball. Draw will either send the cueball into the side or into the point of the pocket. Again, a force-follow might be considered, but George Connor has a better idea: a jump draw. Elevate the cue between 30 and 45 degrees and hit the cueball below center. By making the cueball leave the cloth, it will go forward before coming back. It might not take the path diagrammed (which results from catching part of the rail nose), but you will at least make the cueball go beyond the side pocket before the backspin takes effect. The principle is the basis of many billiard trick shots, but I have never seen it made use of in nine ball, where it would be a handy weapon.

A possible application of jump draw is given in shot 5, Diagram 45. Instead of avoiding a scratch as in the previous example, here the idea is to distort the cueball's path to avoid the 8-ball and draw back to pocket the 9.

Is it possible to cue a ball more than 90 degrees? Willie Jopling claims that it can be done by jumping the cueball and landing slightly on the far side of the object ball.

Two balls are on the foot spot, frozen one behind the other. Can the second one be made straight into the corner? Mike Massey does it with a jump shot.

Jump shots, incidentally, are much easier on heavy, fuzzy cloth than they are on the fine, fast cloths like Simonis from Belgium and Granito from Spain. But even on those cloths there is a way of making jump shots easy while at the same time protecting the cloth from burn marks. The secret is great for trick shots but useless in competition. Needed is a small piece of pool or billiard cloth leftover from the last time your table was covered. It can be as small as a dime. Put it under the cueball, explaining that it will protect the table (which it will). Now see how easy it is to jump all the way over an interfering ball!

Jump shots are also easier to make with a light cue because it tends to bounce off the cueball and not interfere with it. It is common at professional tournaments these days to see players take out a short, light cue when they want to jump over a ball. Sammy Jones, perhaps the foremost practitioner, can jump over a ball when the cueball is less than two inches away from it. Nick Varner sometimes uses just the shaft of his cue when he has to get the cueball off the table in a hurry. The main feature of a jump cue is its light weight, not its short length. A shaft, for example, weighs only four or five ounces, which is an ounce or two less than a cueball. A cue lighter than the cueball will rebound on impact instead of following through.

In games, a jump shot can sometimes be used with devastating effect when breaking clusters apart. Diagram 46 shows a straight-pool position. The break shot is straighter than the player intended; follow will only send the cueball lightly down the side of the pack with little chance of breaking any balls loose. A downward stroke, however, might make the cueball land *on top of* the pack, in which case there almost certainly will be several balls broken free.

Something similar is in Diagram 47. Follow on the cueball might send it off the 4 or the 7 into the corner for a scratch. Even without a scratch,

Diagram 46. Jump shots

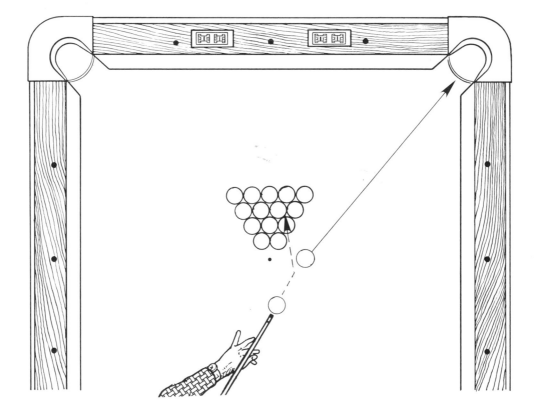

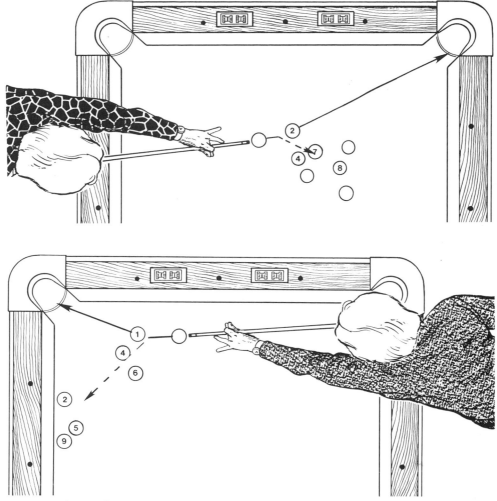

Diagrams 47 and 48: Jump shots

little force can be transferred into the cluster. A better option would be to get the cueball in the air so it climbs over the 7-ball.

Look at Diagram 48. What would you do in a game of nine ball? One possibility would be to make the 1 and stun over to the 6, then play safe off the 2. Cautious but playable. An aggressive (reckless?) player might try a jump shot here because of the chance of running out. Sending the cueball over the 4 and 6 and into either the 2 or 5 will almost certainly leave a way of continuing the run.

I don't mean to imply that jump shots of this sort are easy, but they are not beyond the reach of average players willing to practice. The trick is to hit hard enough to clear the interference, but not so hard to bounce off the table.

Diagram 49 is presented as a puzzle. The game is nine ball. The 8-9 combination is dead, but there seems to be no good way to drive anything

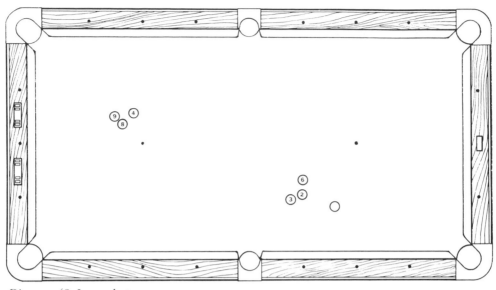

Diagram 49. Jump shots

into it. A safety off the left side of the 2 is what most players would shoot. Don't read the next paragraph if you want to look for another shot.

It's possible to win the game in one stroke. Elevate the cue to about 40 degrees and shoot straight toward the 2. Don't shoot so hard that the cueball jumps over the 2 without touching it; the idea is to hit the top part of the 2. If done right, the cueball will continue down the table and make the combination.

What if the 8 and 2 are interchanged in Diagram 49? Then, of course, you would want to leap over the 8 without touching it, not easy even for top players.

Students interested in other ingenious applications of jump shots and who have *Byrne's Standard Book* should check the diagrams on pages 127 and 128. In *Byrne's Treasury of Trick Shots* there is a whole chapter on jump shots, plus little-known examples on pages 132, 259, and 262.

New and Unusual Trick Shots

In 1981 I was devoting all of my time to collecting trick shots. In my effort to look under every stone, I attended Richie Florence's tournament at Caesar's Tahoe with the intention of picking the brains of every top player I could get my hands on. To encourage them to show me their pet shots, I demonstrated a few curiosities I had picked up from nineteenth-century books on the game plus shots I had invented myself.

The strategy worked well and I had productive sessions with George Middleditch, Mike Massey, Pete Margo, Nick Varner, and other knowledgeable players.

One shot I showed, which I had invented only a month before, has become known as the Penny Wrapper Shot. It's unusual, easy, eye-catching, and amusing. I knew I had found something good when I stumbled across the concept, because trick shots like that are scarce, but I was amazed at how fast the shot sped around the country.

Go to a bank and get two penny wrappers—the paper tubes used for rolls of pennies. Cut one to a length of two and a half inches, which is just longer than the diameter of a pool ball. Use the tubes to tee up two object balls so that they overlap each other, as shown in the enlarged inset in Diagram 50, and put them in the center of the table so that they are aimed at the opposite pockets. When you shoot the cueball under them, knocking the tubes aside, the balls drop straight down, collide, and scurry into the pockets. In the diagram I show the cueball knocking in a third ball; of course it is possible to make the cueball do something more heroic than pocketing a single ball, but I feel that would detract from the central idea. A nice feature of the shot, in addition to its almost dead certainty, is that spectators have no idea what is going to happen until it does. Shoot hard, because the balls must drop straight down.

Whether or not the many fine players who have added the Penny Wrapper Shot to their repertoires have come up with any variations I don't know, but in my trick shot book I explain a dozen shots of the same type,

Diagram 50. Trick shots

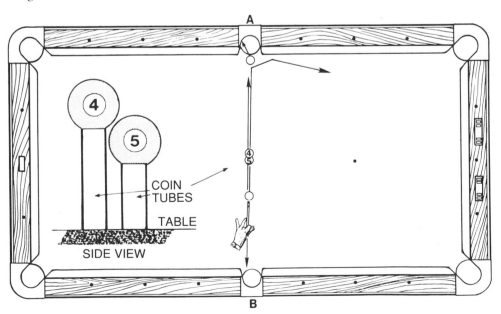

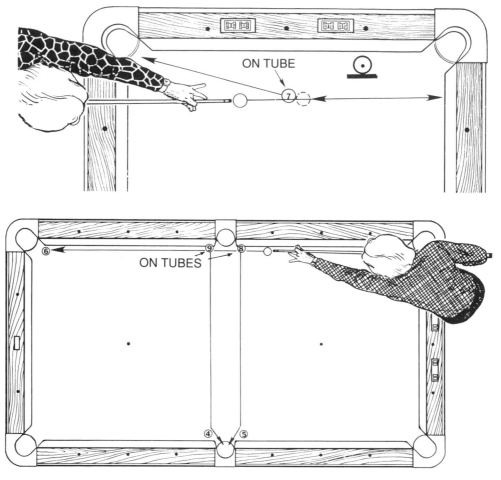

Diagrams 51 and 52: Trick shots

most of which are my own and have never been demonstrated. Here are two of them.

Place the 7-ball on a tube in the center of the table six inches from the end rail (see Diagram 51). Place the cueball so that a line of aim perpendicular to the side rail would pocket the 7 if it were not elevated. If you can shoot under the 7 without English, the 7 will drop straight down and be pocketed in the left-hand corner pocket by the cueball rebounding off the rail. The dashed circle is the rebounding cueball at the moment of impact. To make it easier, elevate two balls on tubes, putting the second one in the position of the dashed circle. It's easy to make the 7 on a combination.

A different idea is illustrated in Diagram 52. If a paper tube with a ball atop it is placed against a rail, then when the cueball removes the tube the elevated ball will drop onto the nose of the cushion and will be sent straight across the table. My use of that discovery is shown. Shoot under two balls and pocket a ball in the left corner with the cueball. The two elevated balls cross the table, one a little later than the other, and follow each other into

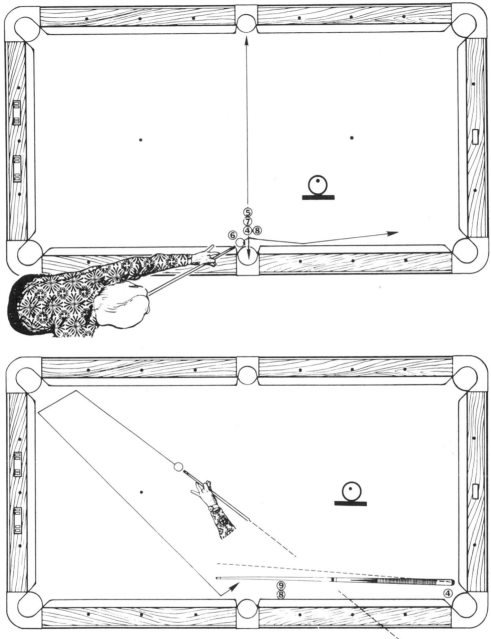

Diagrams 53 and 54: Trick shots

the side pocket after caroming off the two "bumper" balls. The action will come as a surprise even to expert players.

Diagram 53 is a shot I have shown only to a few trusted friends. The 4-ball is the one closest to the side pocket. Who could guess that it can be pulled back into the side from the given position? Use high follow and hit the 4 a hair less than half full. Because the 4 is supported by three balls it can be made to pick up enough reverse English from the spinning cueball

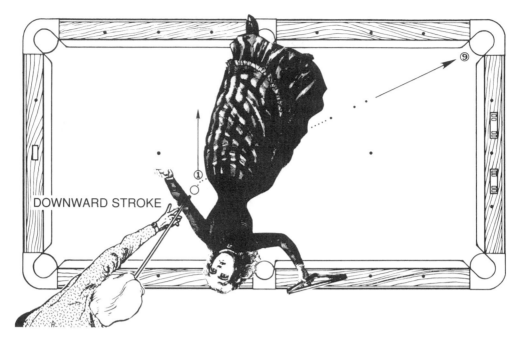

Diagram 55. Trick shots

to make it trickle the few inches that separate it from the pocket. It doesn't seem possible.

Diagram 54 is my adaptation of a billiard shot well known in Japan. From the given position announce that you will pocket the 4-ball (lower right) without jumping over the cue, knocking it in with the cue, or touching the other two balls. The solution is a three-cushion bank. The cueball realigns the cue just enough so that it is guided around the two interfering balls and down the side of the cue into the 4. A clever idea.

The shot in Diagram 55 is so old it has almost been forgotten. Put a victim on the table and with an elevated cue jump the cueball off an object ball so that it hurdles her and pockets a ball in the corner. The main problem is finding a victim who will let you practice until you get the hang of it.

Coping with the Heavy Tavern Cueball

Having grown up on 4½-by-9-foot tables in Dubuque, Iowa, I've never been comfortable playing on anything smaller. One problem I have is philosophical: I tend to think that the smaller the playing surface, the more trivial the game. Marbles and tiddlywinks are never on television, while snooker, played on a gigantic 6-by-12-foot table with tight pockets that present the players with a truly awesome challenge, threatens to devour the world from its power base in England. Maybe our game would be better for television if the major championships were played on 5-by-10-foot tables, as they were 50 years ago. There were compelling commercial reasons for dropping the size of pool tables to 4½-by-9 and then to 4-by-8 and to 3½-by-7, but providing a true test of top-class skill was not one of them.

Another problem I have is adjusting to a cueball that is not the same size and weight as the object balls. Playing on a table smaller than normal is in many ways easier, but the big cueball creates certain difficulties . . . and opportunities.

Rail shots. Making a ball that is frozen to a rail is harder when the cueball is larger. You can see why in Diagram 56. If you hit the ball and the rail at the same time, the line of centers (dotted line) is at such an angle to the rail that the shot will fail unless the pocket is generously wide. As I have explained, cut shots to a ball frozen to a rail require either outside English (in this case, left) to eliminate friction between the balls or hitting the rail slightly first. On a coin-op table, you'd better make sure you are doing one or the other, or both, especially if you have to run the object ball down the long rail past the side pocket.

Cut shots. Some players aim cut shots by imagining where the cueball will be at the moment of contact with the object ball and then aiming the center of the cueball at the center of the imaginary ball. If you learned to do that on regulation equipment, then you might have trouble with cut shots on coin-op tables unless you remember to visualize the imaginary cueball as larger than the object ball. Along any given aiming line, a large cueball will reach the object ball sooner than a same-size cueball. In other words, with a large cueball you must aim for a slightly thinner hit. Diagram 57 shows a single aiming line and two cueballs contacting the object ball. Note how the big one is hitting too much ball. (Exaggerated for clarity.)

On the other hand, players who normally aim by thinking of what point

Diagram 56. The heavy cueball

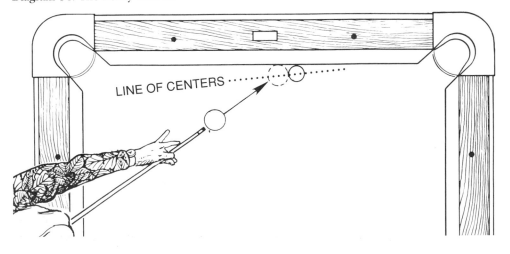

LINE OF CENTERS

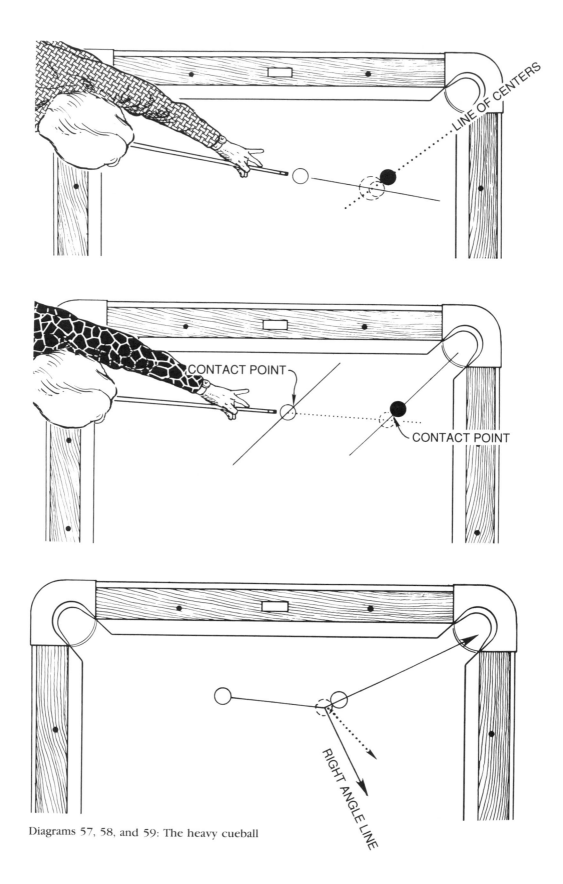

LINE OF CENTERS

CONTACT POINT

CONTACT POINT

RIGHT ANGLE LINE

Diagrams 57, 58, and 59: The heavy cueball

on the side of the cueball must hit the object ball don't have as much trouble with oversized cueballs. Diagram 58 shows how to locate the point. The line through the object ball is the desired ball path; where it emerges from the ball on the side opposite the target is the contact point. Imagine a line through the cueball parallel to the object ball path; where that line intersects the rim of the ball is the point on the cueball that must hit the object ball.

Carom angles. On simple cut shots, the angle the cueball takes off the object ball depends on how much heavier the cueball is than the object ball. (The point can be made dramatically by using a tennis ball for an object ball.) When the balls are identical in weight, the diverging ball paths initially form a right angle. In Diagram 59, the dotted line represents the approximate path that would be followed by a big cueball.

Draw shots. Everybody knows that draw shots are harder with an oversize cueball because it is heavier. Not everybody knows that on draw shots a heavy cueball will advance slightly through the object ball on contact before coming back. That changes the cueball's path considerably and can alter a player's positional strategy.

Consider the shot in Diagram 60. The game is eight ball, and the shooter has the stripes.

What to do? Shoot a head-on draw shot. The opponent's ball will go in on the combination, and the cueball, despite having backspin, will advance far enough to make the striped ball as well before backing up for position on the 8.

Stop shots. A *perfect stop* shot is difficult on a bar table because of the heavy cueball.

Follow shots. Good follow action is easier to get with a heavy cueball, and because of that certain shots which would otherwise be poor choices

Diagram 60. The heavy cueball

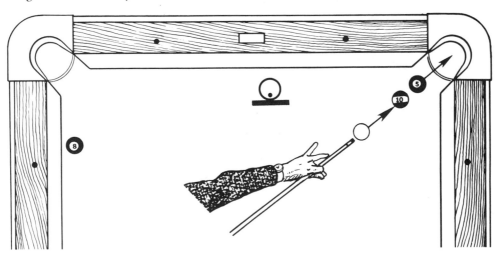

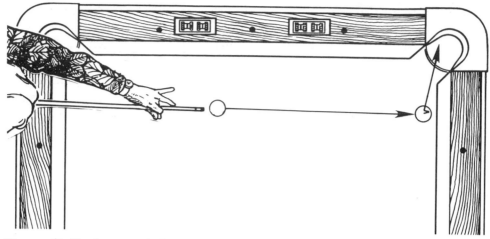

Diagram 61. The heavy cueball

now become eminently feasible. An example is shown in Diagram 61. On a bar table it is easy to double-kiss the object ball into the corner pocket.

I wish manufacturers of coin-op tables had never made the decision in the first place to make the cueball bigger and/or heavier to solve the problem of scratches. Better, I think, would be to eliminate the cueball return mechanism entirely, thus cutting manufacturing costs, and furnish three same-size cueballs with each table. Two cueballs could be lost by scratches during a game without affecting play; whoever scratched the third cueball would be the loser.

Thirty-three Secrets of the Game

That so many top professional players know so little about such things as the coefficient of friction, the conservation of angular momentum, action and reaction, parabolic curves, vector analysis, and angles of incidence and reflection proves that understanding them isn't essential to championship play. But it can't hurt, and it may help. Besides, the physics of the game is fascinating.

Here in summary form are the main assertions I've made over the years in the technical area, leaving out most of the supporting evidence and arguments.

1. The throw effect is most obvious on frozen combinations because the direction of the line of centers can be seen clearly, but it also occurs on simple cut shots.
2. Dirty balls throw more than clean ones because the friction between them is greater. The condition of the cloth does not affect the amount of throw.

3. For average balls, maximum throw is about 6 degrees, which amounts to about six ball widths over the length of a 9-foot table.

4. Maximum throw occurs on a half-ball hit (the angle of approach is 30 degrees).

5. Throw is greatest with very soft speed. Shooting extremely hard reduces the amount of throw by roughly half for angles of approach greater than about 20 degrees.

6. On a simple cut shot, a cueball without sidespin will throw the object ball forward because of friction. To compensate, cut the ball slightly more (make a thinner hit) than geometry would suggest.

7. The throw effect on cut shots can be eliminated by using outside English, which causes the cueball to roll against the object ball instead of rubbing against it. With the right amount of outside English the object ball will travel along a line exactly opposite the cueball contact point.

8. Moistening the contact point between balls almost eliminates throw because it reduces friction to near zero.

9. Chalking the contact point between balls greatly increases friction and therefore throw.

10. The direction, speed, and spin of the cueball are results of how hard the cue hits it, how the cue is oriented in space at the moment of contact, and the eccentricity of the hit (how much off center). Having nothing to do with cueball behavior are such things as the wrist (rigid or flexible), the grip (tight or loose), the follow-through (short or long, straight or crooked), the mental attitude of the player, or body English. Those who believe such things affect the cueball are guilty of voodoo pool. (I'm not saying mental attitude isn't important, only that it doesn't affect the cueball once it's rolling.)

11. Following through is desirable because it is a waste of energy to stop the cue short. After the instant of contact between the tip and the cueball, the cueball can no longer be influenced.

12. A straight follow-through and a snug bridge minimize miscues and help the player hit the cueball at the desired spot and in the desired direction. In addition, a smooth, flowing stroke looks pretty.

13. Sidespin does not significantly affect the angle the cueball takes off the object ball; that angle is influenced by topspin and backspin. Sidespin is used to change the rebound angle and the speed off a rail.

14. If the cue is exactly level, sidespin will not make the cueball curve. To make the cueball curve, it must be struck a downward blow. However, since the cue is at least slightly elevated on most shots, sidespin makes it harder to get a precise hit on the object ball.

15. It is possible to make the cueball curve left with right English. Put the cueball on a piece of chalk on the rail, kneel on the floor, and hit it from beneath.

16. If you strike down on the cueball it will jump . . . unless you trap it under the tip, as in a massé shot.

17. If sidespin is used, the cueball will not initially travel along a line parallel to the cue—it will deflect in a direction opposite the English. The term *squirt* can be used to describe the phenomenon in order to save words like deflection and divergence for other uses.

18. There is less squirt with stiff shafts than with whippy shafts. To test this claim, shoot the "Impossible" Cut Shot (*Byrne's Standard Book*, page 120) the length of the table and keep track of where you have to aim to compensate for squirt.

19. To keep an object ball on the rail on a cut shot, it is best to hit the rail first. Hitting the ball and the rail at the same time will make the object ball leave the rail because of the throw effect. To prove it, set up the rail shot on page 129 of *Byrne's Standard Book* and separate the black ball from the 7 about a quarter-inch. (The correct space depends on the force used and the angle of the cut.)

20. Only a very small fraction of cueball spin can be transmitted to the object ball, but it is enough to make the object ball throw off line by several inches over the length of the table and it is enough to affect the rebound angle significantly on bank shots. The throw occurs at the moment of contact; the object ball doesn't curve because it doesn't receive a downward blow.

21. Because so little spin can be transferred, it is folly to try to make an object ball spin into a corner pocket.

22. When a ball bounces off a rail, the angle of approach does not equal the angle of departure. Methods of calculating banks are not accurate if it is assumed that the two angles are equal. Natural forward roll bends the cueball's path as it leaves the rail, reducing the rebound angle.

23. A cueball struck on its vertical axis seven-tenths of its diameter from the cloth (a hair less than halfway from the center to the top) will have natural forward roll (no slippage between the ball and the cloth). It is almost impossible to get more topspin than natural forward roll, so trying to hit the cueball higher only increases the risk of a miscue.

24. When a cueball hits an object ball full in the face, it will stop dead (see item 33). After stopping, it will follow or draw back, depending on whether it has topspin or backspin. This assumes that the balls are exactly the same weight.

25. A sliding cueball (no topspin or backspin) that hits an object ball full will stop dead and stay there. If it had sidespin only, it will stop and spin in place.

26. On a cut shot, the cueball will leave the object ball along the right-angle line, which is the perpendicular bisector of the line connecting the centers of the balls at the moment of contact.

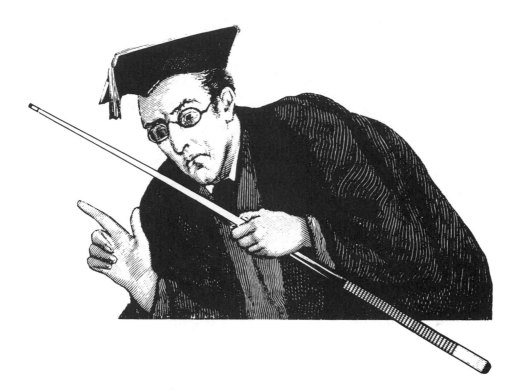

27. On a cut shot, the cueball will bend forward or backward from the right-angle line depending on whether it has topspin or backspin. The curve is a parabola, and its sharpness depends on the speed.

28. On a cut shot, the cueball will stay on the right-angle line if it was sliding (no topspin or backspin) at the moment of contact.

29. On a cut shot, the initial direction the cueball takes forms very nearly a right angle with the direction the object ball takes. To split hairs, the angle is slightly less than 90 degrees because of friction and the inelasticity of the balls. So caroms don't go *quite* along the tangent line.

30. On a massé shot, if you aim through the cueball directly at the point on the cloth that the cueball is touching, the cueball will spurt forward and stop dead. The cue must be elevated to at least 60 degrees. Less than 60 degrees and it is hard to aim at the resting point without miscuing. How far out it goes before stopping depends on the elevation of the cue and the force. Knowing this is very nearly useless.

31. On a massé shot, the direction the cueball ultimately takes is parallel to the line formed by the resting point of the cueball and the point on the cloth at which the cue is aimed.

32. Despite what I say on page 93 of *Byrne's Standard Book* about the "force through shot," draw isn't needed, though it helps.

33. At the instant of contact of the tip with the cueball when sidespin is used, the shaft bends toward the cueball.

34. The best weight of cue for breaking in nine ball varies with the size and strength of the player. Throwing the body into the break shot affects accuracy too much. Timing is the key. That is, making the cue reach its top speed at the instant of contact.

35. Generally speaking, the cueball leaves the tip at twice the speed of the cue. After the hit, the cue slows down to about half-speed.

36. A light cue is better for jump shots because it stops quicker after the hit and doesn't follow through as fast to interfere with the cueball.

37. A cueball with natural forward roll will be deflected most if it hits the object ball half full; that is, if the center of the cueball is aimed at the edge of the object ball. That angle is about 34 degrees for the balls used today.

38. Most of the above depends on having cueballs and object balls of exactly the same weight. Cueballs get worn down and tend to be lighter than the rest of the balls, which don't get struck as often. (Take a scale into a pool hall and see.) In bar pool, of course, the cueball is heavier by design.

Lucky Shots—Ancient and Modern

The shot that gets the biggest response from the audience, that makes the shooter grin the broadest, that makes the opponent hurt the most is the fluke. Forget the long-range cuts, the courageous do-or-die breaks, the sky-rocket power draws, the pinpoint position plays, and the subtle safeties; if you really want to see people whoop and holler, uncork a slop shot.

The injustice of it can be maddening. One player's beautiful run is stopped by a kiss nobody could have foreseen, while his opponent miscues and scores anyway. The best players win in the long run, but along the way we are all alternately battered and bouyed by surprising, even astounding, strokes of luck. All games involve luck, even chess (as when your move makes threats you didn't see at first or counters a threat you weren't aware of), but in pool and billiards it manifests itself in wonderfully dynamic, unpredictable, and stunning ways. In what other game can you try to score, fail, and then score anyway a few seconds later by accident? When it happens, who among us is not moved?

Part of the charm of fluke shots, I think, is that they enable us to witness extremely unlikely events. If the odds against something are a million to one, you can't fail to be excited when you see it happen. I've seen beginners playing eight ball so convulsed with laughter over lucky shots (okay, so they had a few beers) that they could hardly continue the game. The shot gets a greater emotional response than any other and is one of the main ingre-

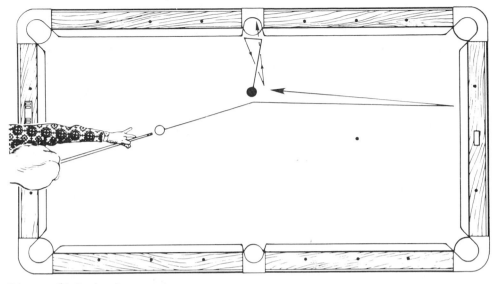

Diagram 62. Lucky shots

dients of the game's charm and appeal. Billiard publications at the turn of the century often diagrammed remarkable accidents contributed by readers, and I think they should again. I have a feeling that a lot of miracles are taking place on the pool tables of this great land without getting the recognition they deserve.

A few years ago, I was watching an eight-ball league match in Novato, Calif. Dr. John Strout, an oto-laryngologist (he takes out tonsils) was playing for game ball. He called the 8 in the side. What happened is shown in Diagram 62. The ball doubled the points of the pocket, rolled out toward the middle of the table, and was cut back into the called pocket by the rebounding cueball. You have to admit that there is something hilarious about this even for those on the losing side.

The most amazing accident that I ever was personally involved in, aside from my own birth, took place on an 8-foot table in a sleaze-bag named Walt & Hank's in Boulder, Colo., in 1954. (See Diagram 63.) My opponent tried to cut a ball inside and at the same time make the 9 in the corner. Well! He missed the ball entirely; the cueball went four rails and then executed the shot as originally planned! For reasons I have never understood, God had reached down and taken my dollar. It was years before I could go back to Colorado.

In pool, a scratch ends your inning; in three-cushion billiards a scratch means a lucky score. Flukes in three cushion have an extra dimension in that they sometimes take quite a long time to unfold. You have time to look at your opponent and watch the blood drain from his face.

A billiard player from Santa Rosa, Calif., named D. Mellinger was faced with the shot in Diagram 64 during a tournament in 1983. He tried to go

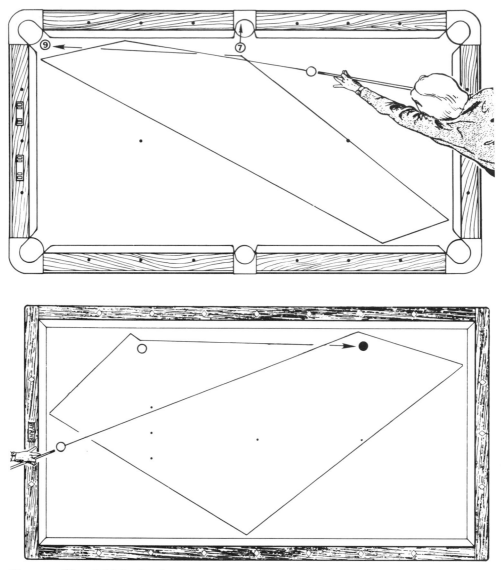

Diagrams 63 and 64: Lucky shots

rail-first off the red but missed the ball entirely. The cueball went around the table and scored in the manner shown. He said he felt terrible about it. More amazing than the shot itself is that during my efforts to find some historical examples I found that the identical accident occurred once before. John A. Thatcher in his *Championship Billiards Old and New*, published in 1898, credits it to one Ben Saylor.

Diagram 65 is also from Thatcher, who says: "A professional, disgruntled and finding what to him seemed an impossible position, shoots hard, drawing Cue Ball with heavy right Twist, taking five Cushions. The Cue Ball meets the red and again going to the Side Cushion effects the Count."

A periodical that presented diagrams of flukes in almost every issue was

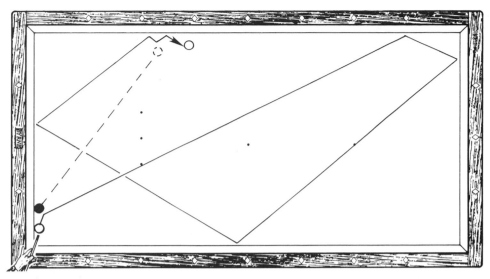

Diagram 65. Lucky shots

The Official Organ of the Billiard Association of Great Britain & Ireland, India & The Colonies, published at the turn of the century. (My thanks to Mike Shamos of Pittsburgh, curator of the Billiard Archive, for sending me photostats.) I haven't reproduced any of them here, though, because they are from the game of English billiards, which isn't played in the United States. One describes a player who accidentally jumped the cueball to the next table, where a point was scored. An example of that theme which took place in Boston in 1945 is described in *Byrne's Treasury of Trick Shots* on page 124.

Note that I haven't described any of my own lucky shots. The reason is that I never make any. I never get a break. My opponents, though! The luck they have is unbelievable!

A Selection of Alternate Games

Players keep coming up with new games, and it's been going on for hundreds of years. Inventors can become consumed by their inventions and go on earnest campaigns trying to bathe others in a heavenly light. I've had to fight off more than one new-game messiah.

Many little-known games deserve more play. Following are a few that languish in rule books or old magazines or that have been sent to me by readers.

A good game for practice or for tournaments is *Equal Offense*, invented by Jerry Briesath, which is straight pool without the safety exchanges. Players begin each inning with an open break and the opportunity to run a maximum of 20 balls. For details see recent editions of the Billiard Congress of America (BCA) rule book or *Byrne's Standard Book*.

Bowlliards, a name to make you gag, is an interesting game that attempts to make use of the bonus scoring method of bowling, which may be part of that game's ungodly popularity. Rack ten balls, bust them open, and start with the cueball behind the line. Using straight pool rules, try to run ten; if you succeed, score it as a strike. If it takes two shots, score it as a spare. If after two shots you still haven't run ten, you get only the number of balls you made as your score for that inning. For more, see the BCA rule book.

The idea of adopting bowling's scoring bonuses is an old one. A booklet published in 1919 by Irvin Huston of Detroit was devoted to a concept he called "Instructive Bowling-Billiards." (There's a catchy title!) Adaptable to any pool or billiard game, the rules require diagrams of ten shots. Scoring on the first try is a strike, on the second try is a spare. Missing twice counts zero and ends the inning.

Honolulu is a game that Kent Andersson likes so much he promotes tournaments for it in his Son of River City Billiards in Anchorage, Alaska. The game is played like straight pool with one huge exception: to count, a shot must be a bank, a kick, a carom, or a combination. First to score eight points wins. Write Kent at 322 E. Fireweek Lane, Anchorage, Alaska 99503, for the complete rules.

Popular in Mexico is a variation of rotation that was called *Chicago* in early editions of the BCA rule book. Instead of racking the balls in a triangle at the start, place them against the cushions a diamond apart, skipping the head rail. The starting layout is given in Diagram 66. The layout in Diagram 67 is excellent for practice because with perfect cueball control it is possible to run all 15 balls.

Kiss Pool. Willie Jopling of trick shot fame is crazy about this and would love to play you for money. It's a heck of a good game. To score, you must pocket the numbered balls by caroming them off the white ball; that is, you use the numbered balls as cueballs. To start, rack the balls with the white ball at the apex and one of the numbered balls behind the line. If you can send the numbered ball into a pocket off the white ball, shoot again, using any numbered ball as your cueball and trying always to "scratch" off the white ball. If the white ball goes in, the inning is over and the white ball is put on or behind the spot. For the full details, see the February 1981 edition of *Billiards Digest*, or write Jopling at P.O. Box 2215, Lynchburg, Va. 24501.

John Furda of Denver has trademarked the name of his game: *High-Cue*. It requires a special set of balls, which will make it tough to popularize, and a tricky scoring system, but a lot of players who have learned it like it, Denver's Danny Medina among them. The rules are in the August 1983 issue of *Billiards Digest*.

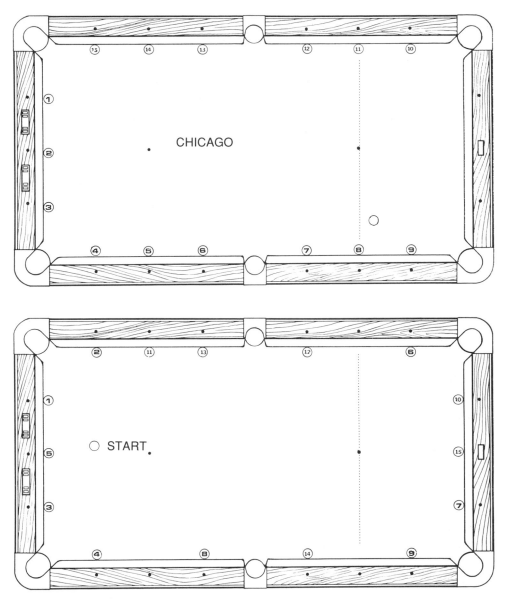

Diagrams 66 and 67: Alternate games

Mayhew. Here's a clever combination of pool, snooker, and poker invented by Barry Mayhew of Canada. At the start, each player takes a pea, the value of which is unknown to the other players. Each player mentally subtracts his pea number from 100 to find the number of points he must score *exactly* to win. Rack nine balls in a diamond with the black in the center. Call the other eight balls "reds." Players alternate pocketing the reds and the black; the reds stay down, the black gets respotted. Making a red counts from one to six points, depending on the pocket. Pockets are valued as shown in Diagram 68. (Barry suggests writing the numbers on the cloth

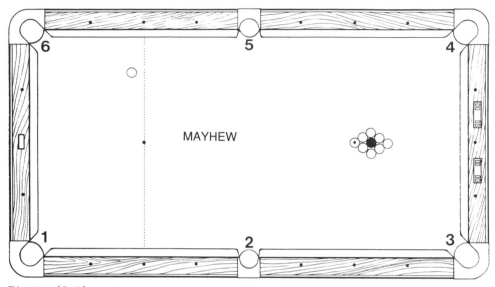

Diagram 68. Alternate games

with chalk.) The black counts twice the value of the pocket. When scores approach 80, bluffing becomes important, for once a player's secret number can be guessed, other players can deny him a shot at his required pocket. As a throw-off, a player might deliberately shoot a ball at a wrong-number pocket and miss. For the full rules, write Barry Mayhew at 2470 Central Ave., Victoria, British Columbia, Canada V8S 2S9.

Stephen Dreyfus likes a game he calls *31 Ford,* which he says is popular in his neck of the woods. Jaw two balls in each pocket and put the remaining three in a line from the foot spot. The idea is to pocket all the balls in the fewest shots starting with ball in hand behind the head string. Since it's within reason to make four balls at once twice, it's possible to make all 15 in seven shots, or with luck, six. A player who misses or scratches must return a ball to the table, which makes a low score harder to achieve than it seems at first. Players continue shooting until they have made all 15 balls or have taken 31 shots. The difficulty of the game can be adjusted by how deeply the balls are placed in the jaws. Says Dreyfus: "Overconfidence and greed frequently result in frustration and defeat." Get the full rules by writing to him at 134 Excelsior Dr., Easley, S.C. 29640.

L. O'Barney Jr., came up with *Barney Pool,* a three-ball game. Put a ball on the head spot, one on the center spot, and one on the foot spot. Starting with the cueball in hand behind the line, try to make the three balls in three shots in the same pocket. (You can't start with the ball on the head spot.) If you do it you get one point, the balls are respotted, and you continue shooting from where the cueball came to rest. For the fine points, write him at Rte. 1, Bailey's Harbor, Wis. 54202.

Here's a really obscure game. It's called *2-Ball*, and it's played only by

George Fels. Put a ball on the head spot and one on the foot spot. The object on each stroke is to hit both balls with the cueball while pocketing one of them. I like it. The rules and some typical shots are given in the December 1982 issue of *Billiards Digest.*

A Selection of Tournament Formats

It's odd the way sports and games are wedded to certain kinds of tournaments. College basketball conferences use the home-and-home double round-robin for league play and the single elimination for postseason play. Tennis is a single-elimination sport. Chess is fond of the so-called Swiss system, in which a tremendous number of players can be accommodated in a few days. Three-cushion billiard tournaments in the United States are almost always round-robins for both preliminaries and finals.

Nine ball seems stuck with the double-elimination format, which is the clumsiest, most confusing, and least satisfactory of all. Golf doesn't even hold proper tournaments—everybody just goes out and plays, and the lowest score wins. The participants don't even have to see each other. (In pool, something similar are Equal Offense events, in which winners are determined by medal rather than match play.)

Following are brief descriptions of the major formats, a word about their pros and cons, and a look at some experiments that should be tried.

The Round-Robin. In a round-robin tournament, every player meets every other player and the one ending with the best record wins. Ties at the end can be broken by playoffs, by total points scored, or by the results of the games already played between the tied players.

It is the fairest format in that there is no "luck of the draw." Players like it because everybody plays the same number of games and nobody gets eliminated.

Disadvantages are that early matches lack tension and that a champion is sometimes determined before the final round. Another minus is that there are always a lot of meaningless games; toward the end, players with no chance at a prize must nevertheless play each other, much to the boredom of the audience, if any.

The concept is simple (all play all), but many spectators can't figure out how to read the wall chart.

The Accelerated Round-Robin. I pushed this variation for years, but my enthusiasm failed to be contagious. The idea is to retain the fairness of the format while eliminating some of the meaningless games. A chart is prepared as if all the entrants are going to play a complete round-robin. At some point during the tournament—the point depends on how many games you want to eliminate—the players with the worst records are dropped. That way the spectators don't have to watch matches between players with no chance at prizes and the tournament as a whole is shortened.

The Blitz Twice-Around. There is another form of accelerated round-robin that I have never been able to sell to anybody, the short-game double elimination. Call it the Blitz Twice-Around. Every player in the tournament plays every other player twice, but to keep it from dragging on too long, the matches are very short. Keeping track is simple: use a standard round-robin chart and divide every square with a diagonal line; the first match result goes above the line, the second goes below. Rather than have, say, ten three-cushion players go through a round-robin of 40-point games, make it twice around with games to 20 points. More excitement and more upsets.

The Single Elimination. This is the simplest and best format for spectators and television because every match is crucial and the precise time of the championship match is known in advance. Spectators are clear on the concept: lose a match, and you're out. The winner is the only undefeated player left at the end. The chart is uncluttered and easy to follow. The reason it isn't used more in pool is that prize funds still come mainly from entry fees. You can't attract enough players if there is a risk of elimination after one round.

The Double Elimination. In this format, you have to lose twice to be eliminated. Winners advance on a chart exactly as in a single-elimination tournament, but losers keep getting fed back in on "the losers' side" of the chart. Casual fans are defeated by the complexity of the chart. Until they lose a match, players are plagued by long waits. Typically, the winner of the losers' bracket (who has one loss) must beat the winners' bracket winner (who is undefeated) twice to win the tournament, even though if he wins the first encounter he has a better record. Television directors hate this format because they can't tell in advance which encounter between the finalists will be decisive. There are ways to get around the problem, but the general public can't be expected to understand the chart.

The Swiss System. Chess tournaments all over the world now use this format, which was pioneered mainly in the United States. Hundreds of players can be accommodated in only a few days and everybody plays the same number of games. To make it work the players, or most of them, have to be accurately rated so that fair pairings can be made. In the first round, the upper half of the field (the highest rated) plays the lower half; after that players with the same won-loss-draw records are matched against each other . . . high against low within the group. Even with 100 or 200 players, after only five or six rounds there are usually only two or three undefeated players left who are playing each other for the title. It works in chess because of the sophisticated ranking system and because players bring their own tables (boards and men). It could work in pool if a lot of tables are available.

The Fullerton Formula. John Fullerton of Mill Valley, Calif., has a table in his house and wanted to host a nine-ball tournament with seven of his friends. Most formats would involve too much waiting between matches. After much discussion, we came up with a format we called the Fullerton Formula, which was enjoyed by all. There are three features. One is short matches—we played races to three. Second is team play—two-man teams compete and partners change for every match. The third is alternate stroke shooting—if you pocket a ball your partner takes the next shot. The result is that everybody stays involved in the tournament, nobody has to wait very long to get to the table, and a good level of sociability develops. Partners discuss strategy and position on each shot because of the alternate stroking. The format is continuous, and the tournament is over when you run out of time. The winner of the tournament is the player who has been on the most winning teams. (See accompanying box for a method of mixing partners.)

The Ladder. Room owners could borrow an idea from chess clubs and keep a continuous ladder tournament going. It never ends. Players are ranked on a posted list. You can only challenge players above you on the list. Your ranking points change with each match you play by an amount depending on the difference in the ranking points of the players. You lose few points, for example, if you drop a match to someone far above you. Handicapping keeps a large number of players interested. Money goes to a prize fund with each match played. Awards can be made monthly.

Mixed Format. Pool promoters should consider the structure now popular in Europe for pro three-cushion tournaments. Start with round-robin

Pairing Chart for the Fullerton Formula

Assign players a letter from A to F. Matches are between two-man teams.

Round 1	AB vs. CD	AB vs. EF	CD vs. EF
Round 2	AC vs. BE	AC vs. DF	BE vs. DF
Round 3	AD vs. BF	AD vs. CE	BF vs. CE
Round 4	AF vs. BC	AF vs. DE	BC vs. DE
Round 5	AB vs. CE	AB vs. DF	CE vs. DF
Round 6	AC vs. BF	AC vs. ED	BF vs. ED
Round 7	AE vs. BC	AE vs. DF	BC vs. DF
Round 8	AF vs. BD	AF vs. CE	BD vs. CE
Round 9	AB vs. CF	AB vs. DE	CF vs. DE
Round 10	AD vs. BC	AD vs. EF	BC vs. EF
Round 11	AE vs. BD	AE vs. CF	BD vs. CF
Round 12	AF vs. BE	AF vs. CD	BE vs. CD
Round 13	AC vs. BD	AC vs. EF	BD vs. EF
Round 14	AD vs. BE	AD vs. CE	BE vs. CF
Round 15	AE vs. BF	AE vs. CD	BF vs. CD

play, end with single elimination. Let's say you have 64 players for a nine-ball tournament. Divide the field into 16 flights of four for round-robin play. Each player is thereby assured of playing at least three matches. The winners of the 16 flights then enter a single-elimination phase. In this way, the last part of the tournament is exciting and easy to follow, yet nobody gets eliminated after only one or two matches. This combination of formats for 64 players would require 111 matches; a full double-elimination tournament would require 126 or 127.

Experimental Formats. I've been tinkering with a format that might attract big fields because there is no entry fee. The idea is that losers must contribute money to a prize fund to continue playing. In other words, losers of up to, say, three matches can buy their way back in. The attraction is that you get to play at least one match before having to put up any money, which should appeal to lower-ranked players. I'm still working on the details. Any suggestions?

Bob Jewett has an interesting idea. Use the single-elimination format, but put the losers into 16-man, short-race, low-entry-fee, consolation tournaments. That would attract players who hate to take the chance of traveling a long way and getting knocked out in the first round. A possibility would be to let the winners of such consolation flights back into the chase for the main prizes, or let them buy their way back in. Something similar would be to modify the double elimination by making losers' bracket races very short until near the end.

How to Argue for a Pool Hall

Want to open a pool hall? Want to expand one you already own or extend its hours? In many precincts you would have an easier time opening a bordello, an arena for dog fights, or a public dump.

It is absolutely amazing how opposed to pool halls some communities are and how differently applications for them are treated from other business proposals. There are cities where the necessary permit is issued by the police department rather than the city council or board of supervisors. There are cities that will give you a permit, but with restrictions so severe you will lose your shirt. (A common ploy is to require unrealistic parking accommodations.) There are cities that will simply say no, get lost, we don't want a pool hall here.

You are in deep water if you want to serve cocktails at tableside. You want to let a person have a drink while he plays pool? Where children might see it? Not in our town! Never mind that the bar down the street has four coin-op tables surrounded by nightly boozers. Never mind that you can have a drink at Gutterball Lanes while bowling with your kids. Pool halls are different. Pool halls are smoky places where crimes are plotted, curses are uttered, and thumbs are broken. We don't want dives like that in River City.

How do you combat such thinking? What do you say to a board of supervisors, no member of which is interested in the game or has ever seen a modern, clean, safe, well-run billiard room? The first thing to do is realize that their fears are not entirely misplaced. A billiard room that is not well managed *can* become a police problem and an eyesore. It will be your job to argue convincingly that what you are proposing is in a different category altogether. You may have to persuade the board to forget the dingy room that once plagued the town as a center for dope dealing, fighting, truancy, and drunks, and to give you a chance to prove that you can provide a recreational center that the community can be proud of. If there is a well-run room in a nearby town, get a statement from the chief of police there or a city council member. If you are a person of exemplary character, stress that. If you have some well-connected local friends, make use of them.

What prompts these remarks is the experience of a friend of mine, Tommy Thomsen. Like many other players, he had dreamed for years about owning his own room. The dream came true in late 1987 when he opened Tommy T's Family Billiards in Beaverton, Oreg., a suburb of Portland. It's an 8,000-square-foot facility with 15 full-size pool tables, three 10-foot billiard tables, and one 12-foot snooker table. Beer and wine are available, but not at the tables. Present Oregon practice forbids, for example, a father from having a beer while he plays a game of eight ball with his minor son. He has to retire to the bar to slake his disgraceful thirst. There is a lunch counter and a separate arcade with 25 video games.

Despite paying some $7,000 for various local fees and permits, Thomsen didn't have permission for the hours of operation he felt were essential for financial success. At first the city council wanted him to close at 10:00 P.M., but an appearance before the planning commission resulted in the right to stay open until midnight on a one-year trial basis. His request for two extra hours on weekends was turned down, which led him to appeal to the council.

Fearing that he wasn't silver-tongued enough to change the minds of the council members, he turned to me for whatever help I might be able to offer. I wrote the following statement and told him he could either read it as an endorsement from me or use it in preparing his own statement.

I make the same offer to readers of this book. If any of my arguments, words, or phrases might help you in an appearance before a commission, council, or board, feel free to use them in any way you see fit. You don't have to give me credit or ask my permission. Change the wording any way you want to suit your style and your particular situation.

Thomsen's request, by the way, was granted, and the council is still happy with the decision.

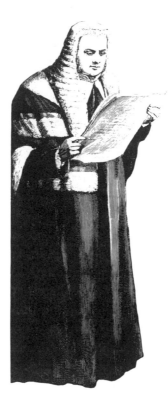

To: *The City Council of Beaverton, Oregon.*
Subject: *Request for extended hours of operation for Tommy T's Family Billiards.*

Ladies and Gentlemen:

Before you is a request from Thomas Thomsen, who asks for permission to keep his new business open until 2:00 A.M. on Friday and Saturday nights.

In ruling on this request, you quite properly must consider its overall effect on the community. The planning commission has recommended that Tommy T's be allowed to stay open until midnight seven days a week. You must now decide whether or not to grant the applicant another four hours of operation a week.

The game of pool, unfortunately for those who love it, is saddled with an image that is as negative as it is unfair. Books, magazines, newspapers, and especially the movies, when they deal with the game at all, almost always show it being played in decrepit public rooms that seem to be halfway houses for the nearest penitentiary. Journalists seem incapable of writing about the game without stressing sleaze. Two popular Paul Newman movies—*The Hustler* and *The Color of Money*—are prime offenders and have gone a long way toward creating the stereotype of the pool hall as a haven for felons, psychopaths, cheaters, con men, drunks, and drifters. As a fiction writer, I can understand the temptation of portraying pool halls in this way, but as a longtime player of the game I know how false is the public perception of the game. The stereotypes have given rise to all sorts of restrictive municipal laws and policies and have interfered with the development in the United States of one of the world's oldest and most popular pastimes. A large segment of the population is being inconvenienced and in some areas even denied a place to practice a wonderful hobby.

How large a segment? Three major surveys by the A. C. Nielsen Company reveal the surprising fact that pool and billiards are second only to bowling in the United States as a competitive participant sport; there are between 20 and 30 million people who play at least one game of pool a year. Americans who want some friendly competition are likelier to pick up a cue than a golf club, a tennis racket, or a ping-pong paddle. And for the first time in its long history, women are playing in significant numbers. In some metropolitan areas, tavern leagues attract a thousand players and more to weekly matches, and as many as one-third to one-half are women.

The growth in the game to such a level has come in spite of resistance and even hostility on the part of many city officials to billiard rooms. The game has been forced to grow mainly by means of coin-operated tables in bars. A bar owner can install a coin-operated pool

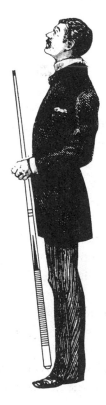

table in most communities with no questions asked as long as he has a vending-machine permit; the businessman who wants to open a billiard room in which players are charged according to how long they play faces one hurdle after another, including the need to make appearances before public bodies such as this one. The difference is unfair and discriminatory.

It is often easier to open an establishment where customers try to get drunk than it is to open an establishment where they merely push balls around with sticks. Why that should be is a question that greatly disturbs players and those involved in the manufacture and distribution of billiard equipment and supplies, a multimillion dollar industry. Certainly there is nothing about the game itself that should raise special fears. Quite the contrary. The game in fact is a wonderful physical and intellectual challenge. It's an absorbing, relaxing pastime, and to play it well takes good eyesight, hand-eye coordination, imagination, concentration, discipline, practice, coaching, and brains. Yes, brains, for to analyze a random array of balls correctly and decide the best way of attacking it can be as complicated as a chess position. The game is also chesslike in its demand for balancing offense and defense. No wonder it has lasted 300 years and is so popular all over the world. In England, for example, a variation called snooker is the number one television sport, far surpassing soccer. To sum it up in a word, the game is *fun*.

Stereotypes must be set aside when dealing with the real world and the issue before you. Certainly there have been and are scary pool halls where you wouldn't want to take your mother or your date . . . unless they were out on bail. And there are billiard rooms that differ from those dens of iniquity as much as day differs from night. What counts, in the end, is the concept and the management. What sort of clientele will the room attract? How will it be supervised and by whom?

A well-conceived and well-managed billiard room can be a civic asset. It can be a bright, open, clean, inviting place that appeals to couples, families, housewives, and seniors—in short, anyone interested in a few hours of congenial social recreation—as well as to serious students of the game. Examples of this new breed of billiard room are springing up all over the country, as the game is enjoying one of its periodic booms. California Billiards in San Jose is one I am familiar with. Star Billiards in Santa Rosa, Calif., is another. Believe me, you can take your mother into either of those places and have a thoroughly enjoyable time. Rooms like those are civic assets because they provide another meeting place, another social focal point, another alternative to the local bar. How many things are there to do in your community on a rainy, snowy, or cold day? A businessman willing to spend money to provide an attractive option should be encouraged and even applauded.

Regarding the specific issue of granting extended hours to Tommy T's, I ask you to look at Tommy Thomsen and his associate, Mort Brock. I can vouch for both of them. I have known them for ten years as men of the highest character and reliability. They are starting this venture because they deeply love the game and because they want to create a place for it that they can be proud of. As lovers of the game, they want to showcase it to its best advantage. I have no doubt at all that Tommy T's Family Billiards will be a credit to Beaverton and to the game. Playing conditions will be so good that I won't be surprised if even some members of this board start chalking up.

The economics of the business, however, require that the facilities be available when customers want to use them. Experience elsewhere suggests that the hours from midnight to two in the morning are often the most popular; in fact, being open during those hours can very well be the key to success of the room. People who have attended a late movie might want to shoot pool for an hour or two before going home on nights not followed by a workday. They might want to play on full-sized equipment in a quiet environment instead of on undersized tables found in bars, and they might want to do it in the company of people more interested in the game than in alcohol.

I urge you, therefore, to grant the petitioner's request for extended hours. Your action will make Beaverton an even more attractive place to live in than it already is.

The Mathematics of Slumps and Streaks

How do you break out of a slump? How do you keep a hot streak going? It's great when you're red hot, in dead stroke, grooved, unconscious, hotter than a pistol, etc., and not so great when you're ice cold, out of stroke, distracted, and unable to hit the broad side of a barn.

The problem of slumps plagues players in all sports and games, and coaches, trainers, the players themselves, psychologists, and gurus of every stripe spend a lot of time trying to solve it. Among the prescriptions are meditation, prayer, legal and illegal drugs, a change in equipment (golfers often credit temporary success to a new putter), psychotherapy, hypnosis, pep talks, sex or avoiding sex, a break from the game, harder or different training, and a return to practicing basics.

I have good news. Many slumps are simply the workings of percentages, odds, and probabilities. For relief look outward toward the impersonal world of statistics instead of inward to the murky depths of your own psyche. You may be doing nothing wrong and nothing may need changing. Recognize that mathematical probability may be to blame, continue playing as you always have, and as surely as day follows night the time will come when you won't be in a slump anymore. You may, in fact, get hotter than a firecracker, which is the same sort of phenomenon. From the point of view of statistics, the difference between a slump and a hot streak is that human beings like one and not the other.

Sports writers are partly to blame for the attention given to slumps and streaks. They are always looking for a story line or a hook, and snake-bit slumpers, unconscious streak shooters, so-called "clutch hitters," come-from-behind teams, and the concept of "momentum" provide them. Evidence suggests that all are fictions.

Take flipping coins, where the odds are even on heads or tails. In 1,000 flips, there is a 62.4 percent chance there'll be a run of ten heads, or tails, in a row. Only 700 flips are needed to give a 50-50 chance of a run of ten.

Or take the spot shot in a game of pool: cueball behind the line, object ball on the foot spot. Let's say you can make it half the time, on average. If the shot comes up once a day, at the end of three years you'll have tried it 1,000 times. The odds are that at some point you'll make it ten times in a row. At another point you'll miss it ten times in a row. In the first case you'll figure you have the shot wired, that you "never" miss it. In the second case you'll wonder what went wrong and start looking for remedies. (If you can make the spot shot three out of four times, then, of course, the chances of missing it ten times in a row are much more remote, approximately one in a million.)

Consider basketball players who make half their shots. Over the course of an 82-game season, a streak of ten shots in a row or a slump of ten consecutive misses should be nothing to get excited about.

A year or so ago psychologists Amos Tversky and Daniel Kahneman studied pro basketball players who tended to make half their shots. No remarkable streak shooters or "hot hands" were found. The streaks that did occur were random and well within chance expectations, just like flipping coins.

Three-cushion billiards serves as a convenient example. By definition, a world-class player averages 1.000 points per inning, which means that he makes a shot and misses one on the average for every trip to the table. In other words, he makes half his shots. If such a player enters a 12-man round-robin tournament of 50-point games, he will take around 1,000 shots. Odds are he will have at least one run of ten, and if you look at tournament charts that's roughly what you find. National champion Al Gilbert's last three-cushion tournament was at the San Francisco Elks Club in February 1989, to cite a case I'm familiar with. Gilbert took the title by winning 12 straight 35-point games. Since he averaged close to 1.000, he took about 850 shots. His high run was nine. The records don't show misses, but it wouldn't be surprising if he missed nine shots in a row at some point. He might as well have been flipping coins. His odds on running nine during the tournament, in fact, were 81 percent; his odds on running ten were 56 percent.

A player who averages .500 is 40 times less likely to step to the table and run ten in three cushion than a 1.000 player. A 1.500 player is five times more likely to run ten than a 1.000 player in any given inning.

George Onoda, a research scientist for IBM in Yorktown Heights, N.Y., who checked the math in this chapter, calculated the odds on a 1.000 average player making runs of various lengths in a 50-point game of three cushion. The player has a 96 percent chance of running five, a 54 percent chance of running seven, and a 9.3 percent chance of running ten. With 1,000 shots, Onoda figured, a .500 player has only a 1.7 percent chance to have a ten run; a 1.000 player has a 62.4 percent chance; a 1.500 player has a 99.8 percent chance. (Omitted from the equations are factors for the tension and pressure that build as the run gets longer.) To run 15 in 1,000 shots, the 1.000 player has a 3 percent chance; the 1.500 player, a 37 percent chance. Knowing these odds may help you win a bet at the next tournament.

Probabalistic reasoning can also be applied to games rather than shots. If you play eight ball with a friend who is exactly as good as you are, and if you play three games every night, then at the end of a year one of you will probably have enjoyed a streak of ten wins in a row at some point. The victim has no reason to think of himself as "a loser." Chance alone explains the disaster.

Of course it isn't *all* predestined. Flaws in technique do creep in and cut a player's skill level, as do health problems, financial and romantic reverses, and so on. Your emotions can rise up and tear you down, no doubt about it, just as they can help you play better than you normally do.

There may be a kind of self-fulfilling prophecy at work. If you lose a few games in a row or miss some shots you usually make, you may believe you are in a slump, tighten up, get nervous, "choke," and find yourself unable to play up to your capabilities. Taking a longer view may help you avoid such self-defeating emotional reactions.

Viewed from the icy, remote peaks of mathematics, slumps can be seen to be inevitable, a simple result of percentages. No need to get depressed or change your game. Just hang in there until the tide turns, which mathematicians call regression to the mean. There is no law that *requires* the tide to turn, but chances are it will over the long haul.

The short haul is different. If you fall several games behind a player of equal ability, chances are you will *stay* behind because the balls have no memory. In an equal contest, you can't afford to spot your opponent anything; both theory and experiments show that in a 50-50 situation, the side that takes an early lead tends to stay in front until the end. What this implies for a nine-ball tournament is that players should alternate breaking. When the winner breaks, the winner of the first game is apt to win several in a row; between evenly matched players, such a handicap is too hard to overcome in a short-race format.

Beware, too, of the so-called "gambler's fallacy." It is widely believed that streaks can be spotted *while they are occurring.* Casinos get rich on such thinking. Crap shooters and blackjack players when they win a few times in a row tend to think that a streak is under way and raise the bet, when in fact streaks can only be identified *in retrospect.* Because cards and dice and pool balls aren't influenced by history, at each step of the way they are subject to the same odds as when the "streak" began and are just as likely to turn against you as before. There is no way to tell if a streak is going to stop or continue. When flipping coins—a pure 50-50 proposition—if a run of nine tails in a row has taken place, the odds of another tail coming up are still 50-50 . . . even though the chances of flipping ten tails in a row are, before the flips begin, 1 in 1,000. In other words, once you've got nine in a row, the odds on ten are 50-50. This assumes, of course, that the coin and the flipping method are fair.

Many books on gambling contain advice on how to bet to take advantage of streaks, to "ride with the winner." If the authors really could tell when a streak is going to lengthen instead of end, you wonder why they try to make money writing books, a long-shot proposition if ever there was one. Casino gambling for such fortune-tellers would be a sure thing.

Another fallacy your emotions might lead you into is generalizing from insufficient evidence. In pool as in life, it is idle to base a conclusion on a sample that is too small to be statistically significant. A couple of years ago I was in a bleachers in Denver, Colo., watching a nine-ball match between Buddy Hall and David Howard. Early on, Hall, breaking with the cueball in the center, twice failed to pocket a ball. For the remainder of the match he broke with the cueball near the right side rail. Later I asked him why he switched and he told me it was because he couldn't make a ball breaking from the center.

In the heat of battle I might have made the same change Buddy Hall tried, even though two successive failures to pocket a ball on the break mean little or nothing. Statistics compiled by Pat Fleming of Accu-Stats show that top players fail to pocket a ball about twice in every five breaks, which is probably oftener than most people would guess. The chances, therefore, of failing to make a ball on the break twice in a row are 4 in 25, or roughly once in every six tries. Three consecutive failures to pocket a ball on the break are a 1 in 15 proposition.

For your homework, write an essay on the following piece of logic: When you take an airplane, the chance is small that there is a bomb aboard; the chance is even smaller—almost zero—that there are *two* bombs aboard. Next time you fly, therefore, take a bomb.

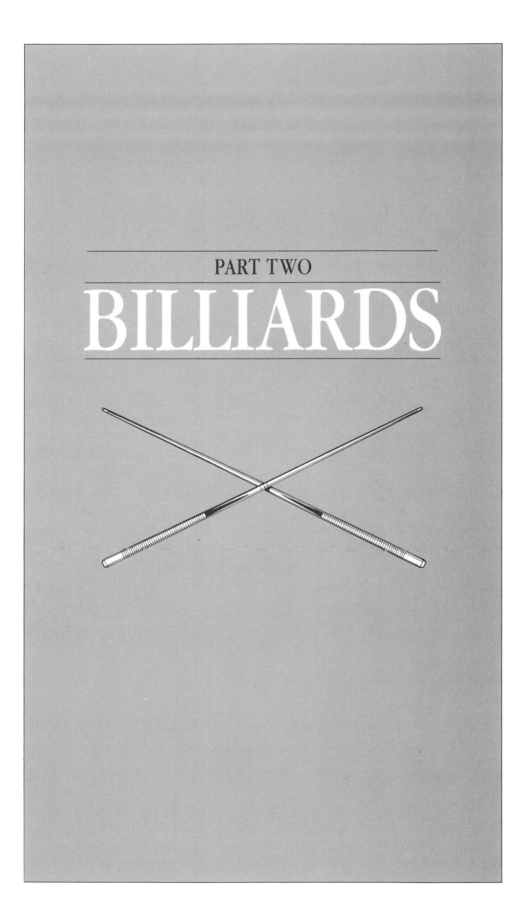

PART TWO

BILLIARDS

A Recipe for Happiness

Take a 5 by 10 ft. table without pockets, cover it with a fine grade of European cloth, add three polished balls, and keep it warm, dry, and well lit for a lifetime. That's a recipe for happiness. There are many splendid games that can be played on a billiard table, but the one most popular in the United States is three-cushion, the subject of this section. The rules are deceptively simple. To score a point, the cueball must hit the other two balls, but before it reaches the second one it must hit three or more cushions. Hidden within that sentence is a wondrous world of spins, curves, and changing speeds, of artistry and imagination.

While what follows can stand alone and serve as an introduction to the game, it is best approached as a complement to the material given in *Byrne's Standard Book of Pool and Billiards*. As in the earlier work, most diagrams include an inset of the cueball resting on the table showing the exact point where the English should be applied.

Warning: Don't try to learn the game entirely from a book. Playing with or at least watching good players is essential. If there are no good players nearby, attend a tournament; for the latest tournament schedule, write to the United States Billiard Association in care of *Billiards Digest Magazine*, 101 E. Erie, Suite 850, Chicago, Ill. 60611-1957.

Eight Easy Shots

A nice feature of three-cushion billiards is that a large part of it depends on knowledge rather than physical skills. Some positions that seem to be difficult or almost impossible are in fact quite easy, *if you know what to do*. As Danny McGoorty once said when I balked at shooting a shot he wanted me to try, "It's so easy that a drunken Girl Scout could make it. All you'd have to do is hold her up to the table."

Let's assume you see a man trying his hand at three-cushion for the first time, floundering helplessly in a sea of ignorance. If he knows nothing about the game, even if he is a halfway decent pool player, he might make no more than one point every ten minutes or so simply because he doesn't notice all the "cookies" lying around. It's agony for me to witness such a spectacle without intervening. I'm always afraid that unless I take emergency action a perfectly fine human being will never experience the joys of the world's most elegant game and will drift in a cloud of discouragement into such things as air hockey and bumper pool.

Let's assume further that the beginner is not too seriously handicapped by his bridge, grip, stance, and stroke and is willing to submit to 30 minutes of instruction. How should the teacher spend that 30 minutes? I think it is best to show how easy certain shots are once you learn to recognize them. The discovery acts as a tonic and another student of the game is born. The frowns of confusion I've seen change into smiles of delight more than make up for the few times I've been punched in the mouth.

Following are a few of the shots I set up for beginners to try. Believe me, it's exhilarating for them to score a lot of points in a hurry.

Shot 1, Diagram 69. The only thing tricky about the ticky is putting the right English on the ball. The ticky is as close to a "gimme" as you can get in three cushion and is a nice gift to present to the student at the start. It's a gift that keeps on giving.

Shot 2, Diagram 70. Rail first. Shots of this type are not only easier than falling off a log, but they carry fewer risks of injury. The point to stress to the student is how softly the ball can be struck. Teach that billiards is a finesse rather than slam-bang game.

Shot 3, Diagram 71. The corner spin out. Doesn't come up nearly as often as the ticky, but helps demonstrate that sometimes the cueball must be driven into a rail with reverse English.

Diagram 69. Easy shots

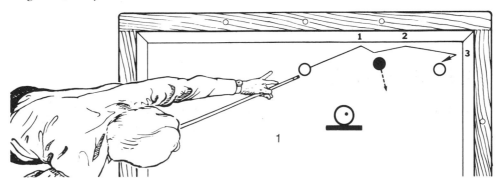

1

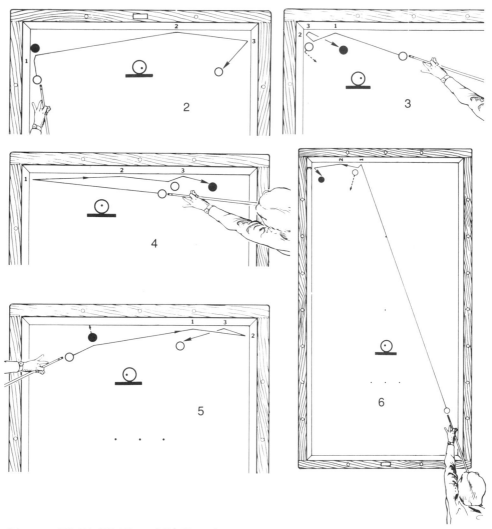

Diagrams 70, 71, 72, 73, and 74: Easy shots

Shot 4, Diagram 72. The backup ticky. No English. Very easy shot when set up like this and one most beginners never think of. Be sure to explain that the first three shots involve running English, reverse English, and no English.

Shot 5, Diagram 73. Doubling the rail off a ball. From what I have noticed about beginners, this shot is about 20 times more difficult than shot 4. If your student misses this four or five times in a row, save him from depression by going on to the next shot, which is *really easy*.

Shot 6, Diagram 74. Long-range ticky. The idea here is simply to show that the shots learned so far have a wide applicability under game conditions. Simply knowing the ticky concept changes this position from a monster into a patsy.

Shot 7, Diagram 75. Doubling the rail is a charming concept to those who have never thought about it before. Pool players, even pretty good ones, almost always fail to use enough English when they first try it. The shot introduces the student to extreme English, which is seldom needed in pool but fairly common in three cushion.

Shot 8, Diagram 76. I throw this shot in not because it's so easy, but because it makes beginners so divinely happy when they make it. It's the well-known draw ticky. Like the previous shot, it satisfies because beginners don't realize that they are capable of such action. Of course they are, but they usually need an instructor's guiding hand to gain the confidence needed to make shots like these when it counts.

Naturally, no opening lesson, not even one lasting only half an hour, should fail to include a discussion of the "big ball" principle and why it is so important in shot selection. Setting up a few shots with the second ball big in the corner is a good way to build a beginner's ego.

In Europe, youngsters start out by playing straight billiards on a small table, then balkline on a small table, then three cushion on a small table, and finally three cushion on the regulation 5 by 10. In the United States, billiard players are almost always pool players first. Teaching a pool player the rudiments of three cushion as suggested here may not make a convert out of him, but at least it will enable him to *watch* a game intelligently.

Diagrams 75 and 76: Easy shots

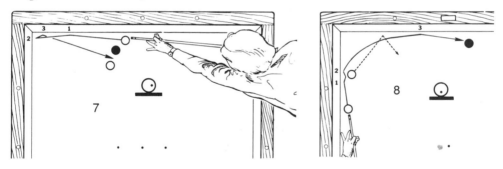

Five Basic Principles

Three cushion is one of the world's hardest games to learn to play well. Not only do you have to know what shot to select, you have to know how much of the first ball to hit, how much English to apply to the cueball, and how hard to hit it. If the student has never handled a cue before, the task is hopeless. Eight ball and straight billiards (no cushions required to score) should be played for a few months first.

Let's say a pretty good pool player asks you for some instruction. Where would you start? Showing him or her how to make a variety of easy shots to build confidence is good, but then what, aside from practice, practice, practice?

Following are five fundamental principles or rules that the newcomer must understand clearly at the outset.

1. **Look for the big ball.** If a ball is near a rail or a corner, see if there is a way to use it as the second object ball, getting all three rails before approaching it, because it is a bigger target than a ball in the middle of the table. In Diagram 77, I have seen countless beginners go off one side of the red ball or the other, maybe because it is closer to the cueball than the white ball. The no-English short-angle off the left side of the red is possible but difficult. Going off the right side of the red and trying for the second and third rails at M and N is slightly easier. Hitting the white ball first, thin on the right side, with the idea of getting the first and second rails at Q and R is not too bad, but not the best available. All three are patterns that must be considered in some positions.

   The best shot, of course, is off the left side of the white with right English. Explain to the student that it is best because the red ball is a huge target, and because the cueball will hit the first three rails with running English, which is the easiest to predict. Fifteen minutes can be spent on this one shot, especially if you also explain its safety and position virtues, considerations that are usually overkill at the beginning.

2. **Go both ways on two-way shots.** If a shot has two ways of scoring, be sure to use enough speed to make it the second way. Even good players sometimes forget this rule. In Diagram 78, the dashed line runs from

Diagram 77. Basic principles

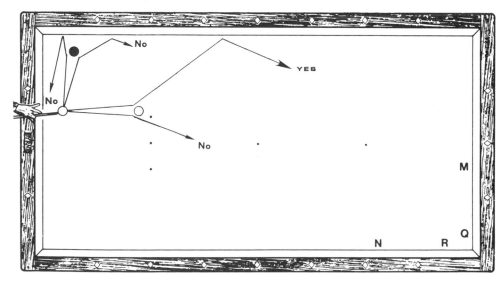

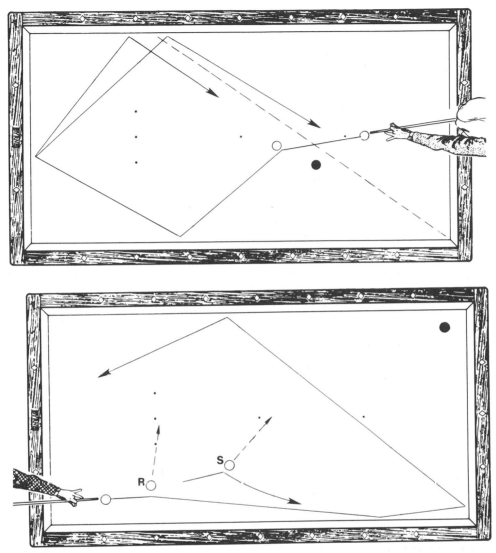

Diagrams 78 and 79: Basic principles

diamond 2 to the corner. Since the red ball is not on this so-called "2-line," the cueball, if it misses the red on the long side after three rails, stands a good chance of hitting it after five. (The shot is not a two-way shot if the red ball is on the 2-line.) In this position the red ball is in fact a big ball, but extra speed must be used to exploit it.

3. **Adjust the speed to the hit.** Don't use unnecessary force. Most shots require precision rather than strength. If the first ball is to be hit thin, then little force is required even on twice-around-the-table shots. Look at Diagram 79. If the first object ball is at R, only medium speed is needed to make the five-rail shot because the first ball can be hit very thin. If the first ball is at S, however, a much harder stroke must be used because

the first ball must be hit half full. An obvious point that many players don't seem to consider.

4. **Choose between the cut and the drive.** Another frequently overlooked concept is that a cueball can be made to carom off an object ball in a given direction with either a thick or thin hit. This means that in many positions the shooter has the option of cutting or driving the first ball. I think the point is worth explaining to students early on. In the lower right corner of Diagram 80, the first ball must be cut fairly thin to keep it from hitting the red. Most beginners would recognize the shot. Few, though, see the similar shot given in the upper left corner of the diagram. The white there must be hit full and banked straight back and forth across the table while the cueball, thanks to high right English, dives forward to almost the same point on the first rail as in the thin-hit version. Beginners rarely see the full-hit option.

5. **Know how the hit affects the spin.** The fuller the cueball hits the first ball, the more linear speed is taken off the cueball; any spin the cueball had to begin with remains almost constant. Thus if a cueball with sidespin only hits an object ball full in the face, it is left with no linear speed at all and spins in place like a top. In practical terms it can be phrased this way: "The fuller you hit the first ball, the more English will be on the cueball."

In Diagram 81, cueball X should be struck with little or no English to make the shot; it will hit the second rail at point X. Left-hand spin is needed to make the shot with cueball Y, which must be made to hit the second rail

Diagram 80. Basic principles

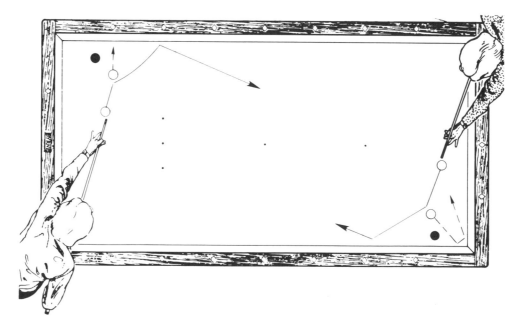

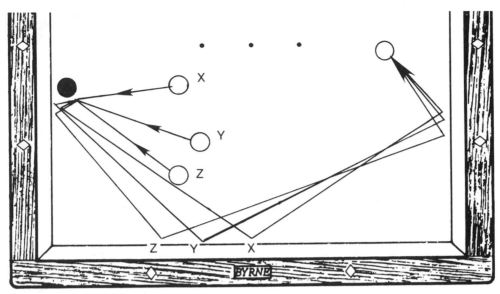

Diagram 81. Basic principles

at point Y. With cueball Z left English is also needed, along with a very full hit on the red ball. The full hit transfers a lot of the linear energy to the red ball, leaving the cueball to travel more slowly to the second rail, spinning much faster than cueball Y. Because of the increased spin, the second rail must be hit at point Z.

Most beginners are surprised to learn that the second rail contact point changes with the starting point of the cueball. But then, beginners are surprised by a lot of things. So are experts.

How Speed Affects Direction

Consider a shot in which scoring is the only goal, not safety or position. In pool, such a shot depends almost entirely on the hit; in three cushion, speed and spin are just as important. Here I will consider three-cushion shots that must be struck fairly hard to have a good chance of success.

Some shots must be struck hard to make sure the cueball reaches the second object ball—force follows, for example, or seven rail backups. In other cases, speed is needed to make sure the cueball doesn't bend forward between the first ball and the rail.

Look at Shot 1, Diagram 82. If the cueball were a few inches from the rail, a little draw would shorten the cueball path enough to score the point. Frozen to the rail (as shown) makes draw impractical. Because the rail forces you to hit the ball with top spin, a hard stroke is essential. The cueball must reach the first rail before the top spin has a chance to bend the path forward

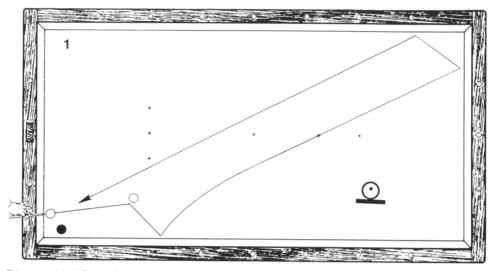

Diagram 82. Effect of speed

any appreciable amount, otherwise the cueball will go much too long. The curve that occurs after the cueball leaves the first rail is okay if the angle off the first rail is sharp enough. Running English makes matters worse. Hit the cueball as close to the center as possible without elevating the cue.

Shot 2, Diagram 83, could be handled as a spin shot with a full hit; as a draw shot with a slightly thinner hit; or as a holdup shot with a still thinner hit and left English. But all of those options have kiss problems. Another way to handle the position is with a center ball hit, striking the cueball hard enough so that it is still sliding when it hits the first object ball. That way you are banking the first ball away from the second one, and you are forcing the cueball to travel in a straight line to the first rail, which is easier to judge than the curving line that would result if the cueball had any top spin. In planning the shot, pick out the spot you want to hit on the first rail and then try to hit it with a straight-line carom off the first ball, and with little or no English.

Shot 3, Diagram 83, comes up frequently. If you use a half-ball hit on the first ball (which gives maximum deflection), running English and soft or medium speed, you will miss the red ball on the short side. The problem is that the cueball will bend forward after it hits the first ball, thus striking the first rail too far from the corner. Of course, the shot can be lengthened by elevating the cue and drawing the cueball closer to the corner, but when you do that you have the problem of judging the massé curve as the cueball approaches the first ball.

The best approach, in my opinion, is to keep the cue as level as possible, use straight right English, and hit the cueball so hard it will not have time to acquire forward spin from the cloth before it reaches the ball. If the cueball is frozen to the rail, thus forcing you to hit the cueball above center,

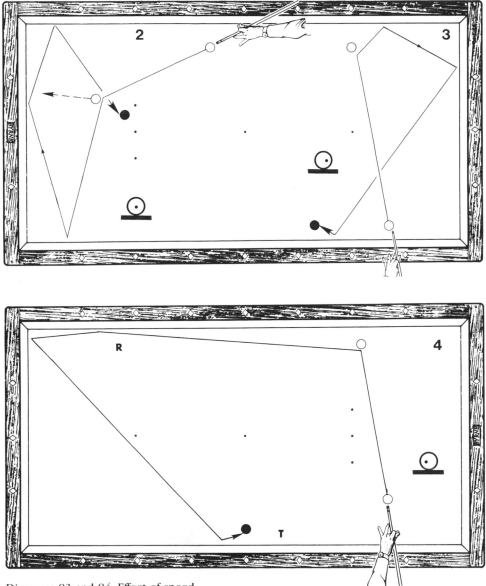

Diagrams 83 and 84: Effect of speed

you must use even more speed so that the cueball will hit the first rail before bending forward.

Take a look at shot 4, Diagram 84. The second ball is lying off diamond 4 and can be reached if the cueball hits the first rail fairly close to the corner. That can't be done if there is any top spin on the cueball. Drawing the cueball off the first ball is a possibility, but then the curve from the ball to the first rail must be judged correctly. Easier is to stun the cueball into the corner as diagrammed, which means sliding the cueball into the first ball. Use straight left English and hit it hard enough so that the cueball has no chance to pick up forward roll from the cloth as it crosses the table. The same technique,

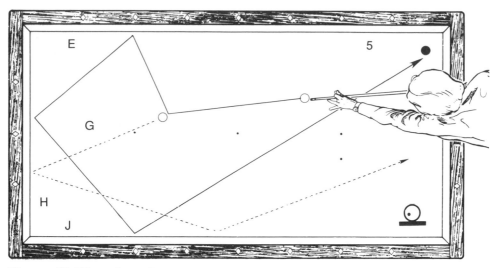

Diagram 85. Effect of speed

except with right English, can be used for double-the-rail shots when the object ball is at R.

A couple of final observations: If the second ball is at T, try some other pattern; the fourth diamond is the best you can hope for without resorting to hard-to-judge, no-English, or holdup shots. Finally, if the first ball is closer to the rail than shown, top spin can be considered because it will bend the cueball forward after it leaves the first rail.

Shot 5, Diagram 85, is a spin shot, but it also fits this group of shots because the need is there to make the cueball travel from the first ball to the rail without the forward curve that topspin would give it. The reason is that a full hit is needed to avoid a possible kiss. Use of running English—sending the cueball to E and the object ball to H—runs the risk of banking the object ball two rails into the red. Hitting the object ball thinner and using draw—sending the object ball to J—is likely to result in a kiss at G.

The diagram shows what happens with a full hit—the object ball follows the dashed line and doesn't disturb the red. The cueball, if hit hard enough, will take a straight line to the first rail, and spin will carry it around the table from there.

Remember when making the shot this way that it is almost impossible to miss it short, so use plenty of spin and hit the first ball as full as you can without killing the cueball completely.

Shots Easier Than They Look

One of the first things a student of three-cushion billiards learns is the importance of the so-called "big" ball. If one of the two object balls is several inches from a rail or corner, it presents a much greater target than it would frozen to a rail or in the center of the table. Therefore, a shot should be selected that allows the cueball to approach it after first hitting the other ball and three or more rails.

Unfortunately, the "big" ball principle can exert a kind of tyranny over the player trying to find the best shot. Sometimes, for reasons of position or safety, or when the hit on the other ball is too difficult, the big ball should be hit first. The subject of this lesson is the *hidden* "big" ball; that is, shots in which one ball is much "bigger" than it first appears.

Shot 1, Diagram 86, is a common example. Cross-table shots of this type, especially when the second ball is a foot or so off the rail, are good choices because of the "two-way" feature—if you miss the red off the third rail, you may get it off the fourth, or even the fifth. Note that I have shown the cueball going into the first rail at a slight negative angle. This is sometimes necessary in order to give the cueball path enough of an angle into the second rail. Without this angle the cueball might go straight across the table off the second or third rail, sometimes even going "uphill" away from the red ball. Slight elevation of the cue, many top players believe, also helps keep the cueball zigzagging down the table toward the second ball. The same shot often comes up shifted to the left, with the red ball at C. It's

Diagram 86. Not so tough shots

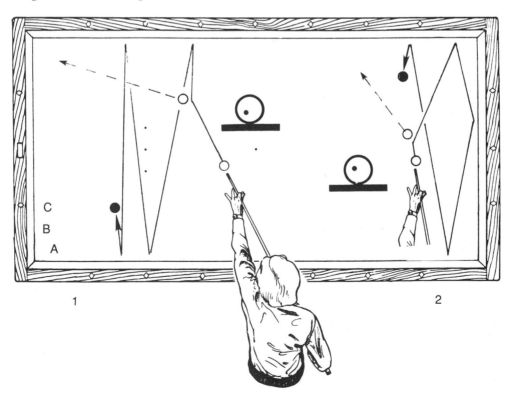

1   2

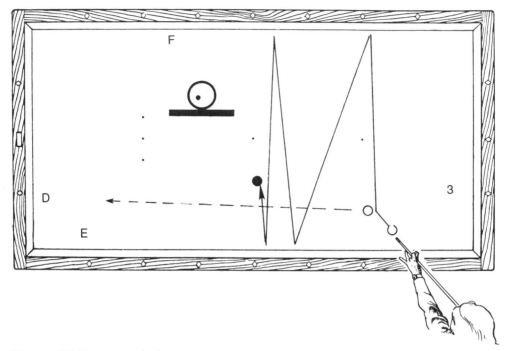

Diagram 87. Not so tough shots

tempting to simply drop the red ball to A and B, but often the second ball is huge if you go across the table one more time.

The same idea applies to shot 3, Diagram 87. When the balls are like this, a cross-table is often overlooked, perhaps because there are usually other good options as well. For instance, there is a four-rail shot, with the cueball hitting the first rail at D, the five-rail shot, with the cueball hitting the first rail at E, the double-the-rail reverse English shot, hitting E first, and the force-follow shot to F. But see how "big" the red ball is in the diagrammed pattern, even though it is a diamond and a half away from the rail. This should be stroked with some authority to be certain you make it off four rails if you miss it off three.

"Big" ball shots can be thought of as two-way or three-way shots. If there is more than one way for the cueball to hit the second ball, be sure to use enough speed to keep all options viable. Danny McGoorty put it this way: "Always shoot hard enough to make the shot the second way. If you can't remember that, get a job."

Now, go back to shot 2, Diagram 86. It is certainly possible to make this shot by going five rails thin off the left side of the white. But when the cueball reaches the fourth rail, the white is liable to be waiting there like a log in the road. The diagrammed shot is an excellent alternative. Even though the red is a foot from the side rail, the cueball can't go through the hole even if you miss off the third rail.

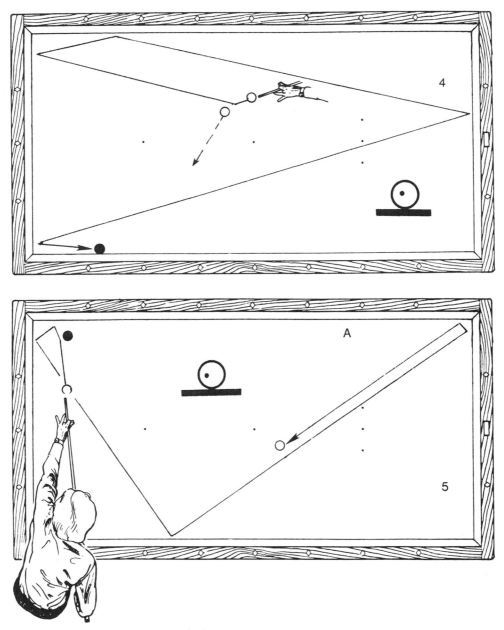

Diagrams 88 and 89: Not so tough shots

In shot 4, Diagram 88, the player can try a chancy cross-table off the left side of the white, or a five-railer off the right side of the white, which would take a strong stroke and draw to get it short enough. In the diagrammed path, however, the red becomes "big" as a house. If you don't make it going in, there is a good chance to make it backing out.

In shot 5, Diagram 89, the red is "big" in the corner, but there is no way to take advantage of it. Drawing the cueball off the white ball to A is possible, but not easy. The educational feature of the diagram is that the

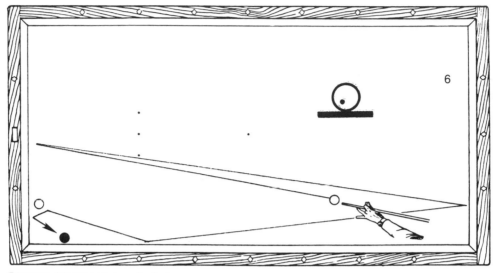

Diagram 90. Not so tough shots

white ball, even though it is near the center of the table, is nevertheless "big." It is just off the cueball track connecting the third rail to the corner, so if you miss it going in, you'll probably catch it coming out. Here you not only have to make sure to hit the ball hard enough to make the shot the second way, you have to know there *is* a second way.

Shot 6, Diagram 90, is a variation on the theme. The two object balls taken together are "bigger" than they seem—provided you find the right way to approach them. The up and down bank shot is by far the best shot in this position because, if you hit the first two rails approximately right, there are several ways to score.

The Time Shot

You have to be aware of certain possibilities before you can exploit them. The best shot, for example, is sometimes the one that requires relocating the second object ball. Beginners almost never see time shots, as they are called, and even intermediates can overlook some fairly easy chances.

The easiest time-shot pattern is the one shown in Diagram 91. There are three fairly good bank shots that can be tried, but by far the highest percentage shot is the one in which the red ball is bumped into the corner, where it becomes a large target. With the balls close together like this, a top player will score the point nine out of ten times. If the two object balls are six inches or a foot apart, the hit on the first ball becomes critical. Usually the player has some freedom in blending hit, speed, and English, but on time

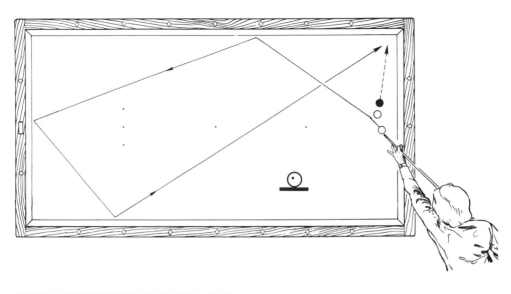

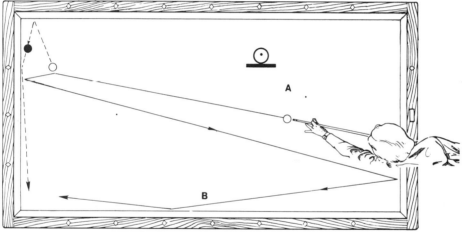

Diagrams 91 and 92: Time shots

shots with separated object balls the hit and speed are largely fixed—only the English can be varied. In aiming, set up to get the required hit, then select the amount of English that will give the cueball a favorable angle off the first rail.

It is usually not necessary to predict the exact spot where the second object ball will be when the cueball arrives; it is more a matter of getting it into an area where the cueball is most likely to encounter it.

The shot in Diagram 92 is admittedly difficult, but so is everything else that might be suggested, including the reverse English cross-table off the white. The time shot has a better chance of scoring than you might think, especially if you can overcome feelings of hopelessness when trying it. Again, it is not necessary to predict exactly where the point will be scored—just bump the red ball to the other side of the table and hope for the best. (If

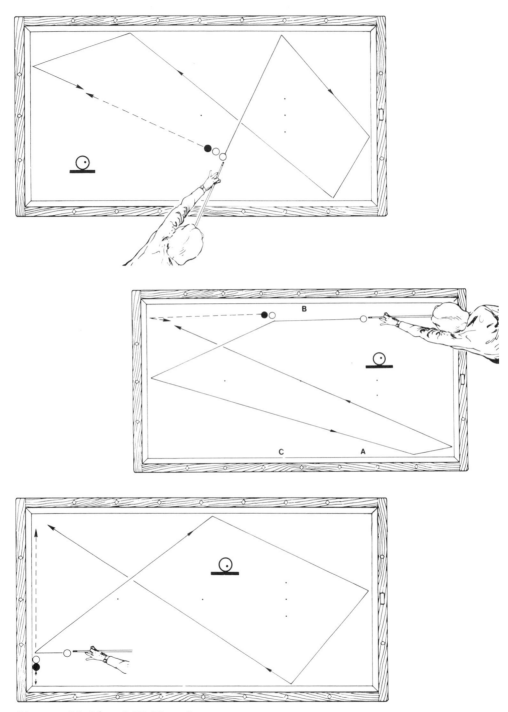

Diagrams 93, 94, and 95: Time shots

the cueball is at A to begin with, go around the table four rails instead of up and down, contacting B on the second rail.)

The greatest time shot I ever saw made in a tournament game was executed by Humberto Suguimizu of Peru, many times champion of South

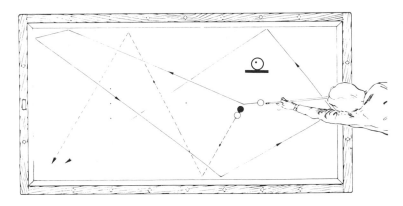

Diagram 96. Time shots

America. Playing at the world tournament in Las Vegas in May 1978, he was faced with the position given in Diagram 93. After studying the shot for several minutes, he played a five-rail backup time shot, scoring it as drawn. The concept was as remarkable as the execution.

The best time shot I ever made in a game appears in Diagram 94. The position came up in an April 1979 match against Pepe Gomez, former balkline champion of Mexico, at Tiff's Billiards in North Hollywood, Calif. A thin hit was required to keep the red ball from traveling more than a few feet, and a touch of holdup was applied to the cueball to make it rebound steeply off the first rail. The shot was feasible only because the two object balls were within a half-inch of each other. Had they been, say, three inches apart, the cross-table bank (three side rails) might have been a good choice, using right English to make the cueball hit A, B, and C before approaching the balls.

The four-rail time shot in Diagram 95 is not difficult and was often a part of former world champion Welker Cochran's exhibition program. The first ball must be hit quite thin so the red doesn't pick up too much speed. The reaction this shot gets from spectators is not deserved.

Another not-too-difficult shot from the Cochran repertoire is given in Diagram 96. The cueball goes five rails around the table, the second object ball goes twice across. You'll have to experiment with this one to discover the exact placement of the balls to suit your table.

The Kiss-back Shot

Kissing the cueball back off a ball frozen to a rail is another idea that seldom occurs to beginning three-cushion players. Kiss-back opportunities may not arise for hundreds of points; then several may crop up in a single game. The pattern is common enough that every student should devote some time to learning the angles, English, and speed required.

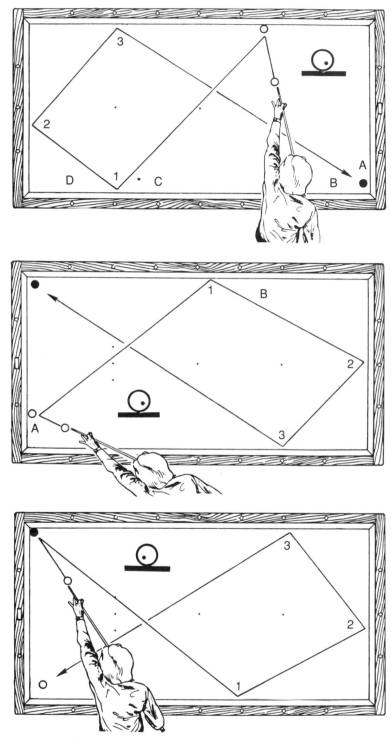

Diagrams 97, 98, and 99: Kiss-back shots

The commonest application of the theme is given in Diagram 97. The main thing to remember in shots of this type is to hit the cueball below center—draw contributes to cueball speed on the rebound and holds the cueball's path straight. Follow slows the cueball down and bends its path.

In the diagram, note that low *right* English is applied so that the cueball will contact the three required rails with running English. (English that makes the cueball speed up on hitting a rail is called running. The opposite is holdup or reverse.)

If the red ball were at point a in the diagram, it would be best to kiss back to point c and finally to the fourth rail at point b. The reason is that the fuller the hit on the frozen ball the easier it is to judge the rebound angle. A four-rail shot kissing back to c is easier, therefore, than the three-rail shot kissing back to d.

Another standard application is given in Diagram 98. Again, remember to use low English. If the first ball were at a, it would be better to try a thin hit off the right side of the ball instead of a kiss-back. Not only is the thin hit (provided it isn't too thin) easier to judge, but the first ball is likely to end up in the vicinity of b, providing a good second shot.

There are other reasons for favoring the thin hit over the kiss-back when a choice is presented. The thin hit in this position requires less English, less chance of a miscue, and no need to estimate the curve of the cueball on its way to the frozen ball.

In Diagram 99, twice-across off the white must be considered, but if the red is frozen in the corner the kiss-back is by far the best choice. In fact, with the white "big" in the corner, the kiss-back is sometimes the highest percentage shot even if the red isn't frozen.

In Diagram 100, some players might go for the short-angle with right English off the left side of the red. The trouble with that shot is that it is hard to reach for a right-hander, it is a sellout if you miss, and the red might bank into the second object ball before the cueball gets there. Kissing back off the white as drawn is frequently the best idea. You'll have to try it a few times to get a feeling for the hit required.

Diagram 100. Kiss-back shots

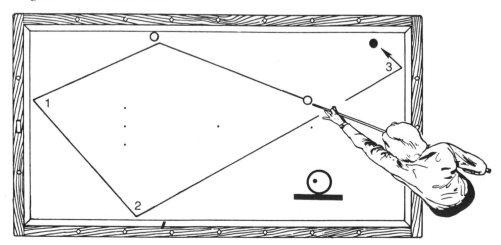

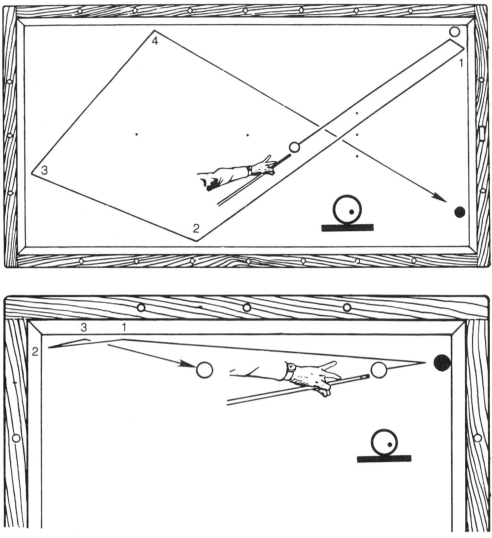

Diagrams 101 and 102: Kiss-back shots

In positions similar to the one in Diagram 101, twice across off the white or four rails off the left side of the red might be the best shots. If the white ball is frozen, as in the diagram, the four-rail kiss shot should be considered as well. A little-known shot, and by no means easy.

A beautiful example of the pattern is given in Diagram 102—kiss-back through the hole and double the rail out of the corner. Make this in an important game, or any game, and you'll feel good for weeks.

The Principles of Defense

Good defensive strategy, absolutely essential to winning in three-cushion billiards, is hardly ever mentioned in the scanty literature of the game. Willie

Hoppe was justly famous for his defensive skills, yet in his 1941 book on how to play the game there is not a single line or diagram devoted to safety play.

Defense in billiards consists of far more than simply playing "easy to up the red" and its corollary, "hard away from the white." Knowledge and experience are involved in knowing which of several shots and stratagems to pick in given situations. Often an exquisite control of speed is required. A player's personality is a factor—is he a confident daredevil willing to throw caution to the winds in an attempt to score, or is he a chicken who protects himself at all costs? If faced with ten tough leaves in a row will he lose his patience and take unneccessary risks?

It is a simple matter to leave your opponent's cueball at one end of the table and two object balls at the other. The trick is to do that and still make the point or come close to making it. On many shots it is necessary to distort the standard cueball path slightly, thus adding difficulty to the shot, in order to make sure you don't leave anything easy. Each player must decide for himself when he steps to the table whether he should ignore defense and try to make the shot, whether he should play position instead of safe, and how much he should reduce his chances of scoring for reasons of self-protection.

Some general rules: Don't die too close to the red or you'll leave a decent bank. Forget safety play on "big ball" shots and standard naturals. Watch out for shots that result in tickys if you miss. Don't relax on shots that have a safe leave built into them—try hard to score. Early in the game, or if you are hitting the ball well, ease off on the safety play and try to bury your opponent with points. Late in a close game, or if you are not playing up to par, hang on and hope for a miracle by leaving your opponent nothing.

Out of literally hundreds of positions that could be discussed, I have chosen only six. (For more on this vital subject, see pages 276–280 of *Byrne's Standard Book.*)

The easiest way to make the shot in Diagram 103 is with a half-ball hit, which banks the white ball to the sellout end of the table. To avoid that, there are two hits to think about in positions of this type: thick and thin. A feather-thin hit, cutting the white toward point c, with maximum right English to put the cueball on a scoring path off the first rail, will leave your opponent far from his work if you miss. Or you can hit the white full with follow and slight right English, banking the white to point b and back to c. In both cases the cueball can be made to die near the red.

In Diagram 104 the shooter has the choice of using right English with slight draw to score on the red off three rails, or using natural running English for a four-rail shot as diagrammed. This way is best because the white ball is cut slightly thinner, thus making sure that it will be banked to the short rail near a. Banking the white to a rather than b is the key to a safe

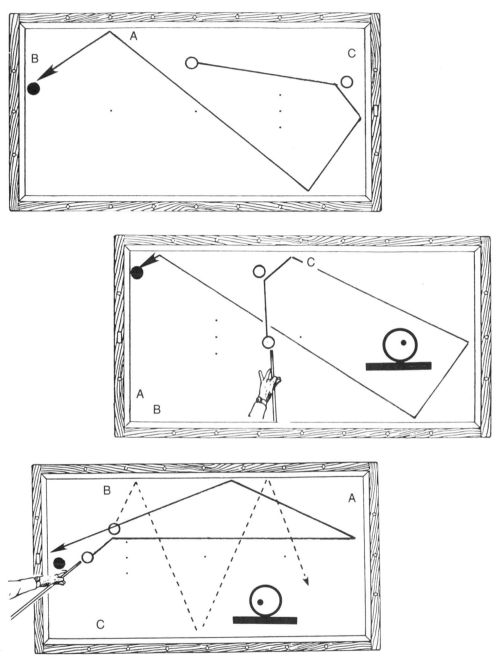

Diagrams 103, 104, and 105: Principles of defense

leave as well as to position, for if the white hits a and b and ends up near c you will be in perfect shape.

The shot in Diagram 105 is a little subtler. Most beginning and intermediate players would simply hit the white thin, trying to make the cueball hit the first rail near a. The trouble is that the white gets banked from b to c and will be close to the red, at least, if you miss. Better here is a soft spin shot. Hit the white fairly full with maximum left English. The white travels

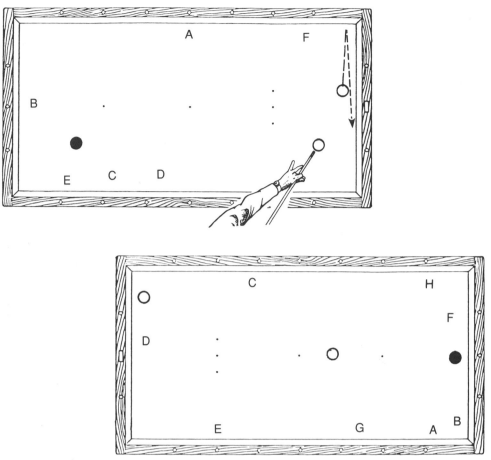

Diagrams 106 and 107: Principles of defense

at moderate speed to the first rail spinning like a top, following the diagrammed path, stopping near the red if you miss. The white is zigzagged down the table as shown. Spinning the cueball is also good here because it enlarges the target on the third rail.

Most players would know enough to go off the white in Diagram 106, but how many know that, other things being equal, it is better to draw back and hit the second rail at e than it is to use left English and hit the second rail at a? The reason is that if you follow the a-b path and you miss, stopping near c or d, you stand a good chance of leaving a ticky. The white ball, of course, is banked straight across to make sure it stays at the right end of the table. If the cueball were a little farther to the right it might be possible to hit the second rail at f and the third rail at c. That would be good from a safety point of view, because if the cueball goes past the red without hitting it, it travels still farther away from the opponent's cueball.

In Diagram 107 the cueball is at the left end of the table. What's the best shot? It might be possible to go off the right side of white (the so-called cross-table shot), contact the first rail at g and the second rail at h, and bank

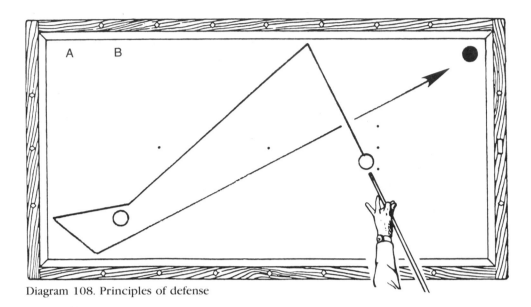

Diagram 108. Principles of defense

the white down to c or d for a safe leave. Another idea is the five-rail bank (a-b-c-d-e), clipping the white and then the red. The sneaky part is to make sure you play the bank *long* and with just enough speed so that if you miss the white the cueball ends up around f. Depending on the position, the five-rail bank might be best the other way, hitting the first rail at c. There are many other banks where the balls are spread far apart in which a slow speed will leave the cueball far from the white.

The last shot, Diagram 108, is something for the experts to ponder. I can't imagine an American player trying it, with the possible exception of Carlos Hallon, who has several similar shots in his repertoire. It was shown to me by Abel Calderon, genial proprietor of the beautiful Abel's Club in Astoria, N.Y., who saw it played in a South American tournament. A nice feature is that not only is the shooter protected if he misses, he is liable to have position if he scores, as the white might end up near b. What other shot is there? Well, okay, you could draw straight off the white with left English to the first rail at a, but not many of us are Zeke Navarra.

The Basics of Position Play

Many if not most casual three-cushion players spend their lives without ever trying to leave themselves an easy shot. They think ahead in that they try not to leave the other guy anything. But play position? Never. Newcomers to the game, in fact, are often surprised to hear that position play is even possible in a game that seems so formless and abstract.

The best players in the world, on the other hand, especially Raymond

Ceulemans of Belgium, at least *consider* position on the majority of shots. When faced with a relatively easy shot (one in which the second object ball is "big" in a corner, for example) even weak players are foolish if they don't try to set themselves up. The better the player, of course, the more shots are *relatively easy*.

The position player in billiards is often not trying to leave himself a specific shot. Instead, he is trying for an arrangement of the balls that awareness of a few principles tells him will more likely present a makeable shot than if he had relied on chance alone. Playing position doesn't necessarily make the shot harder. It is often just as easy to hit the object ball full with extra English as it is to hit it thin, just as easy to hit it soft as hard. In one case you may be playing yourself safe and in the other setting yourself up. When faced with one or more shots of roughly the same difficulty, the position player picks the one that contains both position and safety elements, while the less-informed player thinks of safety alone.

On some shots, trying for position reduces the chance of scoring, but the risk may be worth it in view of the reward. Position play in three cushion often requires leaving the cueball close to the second object ball—say, within a foot—otherwise the possibilities are too great to calculate. Further, it requires leaving the first object ball not in an exact spot but in a certain area of the table. The desired position zones for the first object ball are quite large, which means that position play is not as hard as neophytes might think.

Take the position in Diagram 109. The red ball is *big* in the corner, and with cueball a, this is a very easy shot, thanks to the size of the final target. An easy position pattern calls for driving the first object ball along the dashed path so that it ends up in the shaded zone, while at the same

Diagram 109. Position play

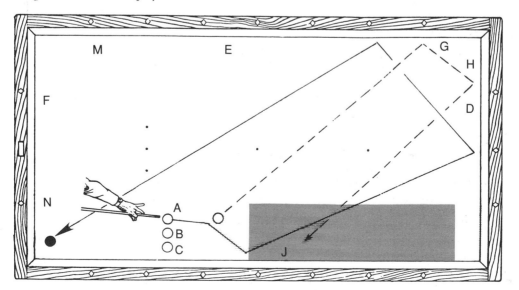

time making the cueball land softly on the red. If both of these ends are accomplished, there will be another good shot the great majority of the time.

But what if the cueball is at point b? Now, if you drive the object ball along the same dashed path the cueball will run along, hitting the fourth rail near n, and the shot will be missed. If you compensate by using a little draw on the cueball to bend it back into a scoring path, then too much speed is needed and the white ball will go into the shaded zone and back out again. A good position play using cueball b would be to drive the white into the short rail at d, then to e and f and back into the shaded area. Since the white will be entering the position zone more or less lengthwise, there is a considerable margin of error. Not quite as promising, though sometimes the best bet, is to hit the white rather thin with draw, banking it twice across to the upper right corner near h.

With cueball c, the first two patterns are out of the question. The white still can be put into the shaded position zone, though. Drive the white into the long rail at g, sending it five rails (g-h-j-f-m) and back into the shaded area. To make the point the cueball has to be hit with low left, drawing it with spin into the first rail near j. The cueball can be made to land softly on the red from all three starting points. (For more examples, patterns, and discussions of position play, see *Byrne's Standard Book*, pages 286–297.

Former national champion Eddie Robin, who has made special study of position play, identifies four classes of leaves. Best of all, he says, is leaving all three balls in a rectangle no bigger than, say 1 by 2 diamonds, especially if no ball is near a rail. Next best is leaving the first ball within a foot or two of the center of the table, especially if neither of the other two balls is near a cushion. Third is leaving the three balls near the same long rail, especially if the cueball is between the other two or close to one of them. (The shots discussed in the first part of this discussion fall into this category.) The fourth and least desirable class of shot is when one object ball is near a corner and the cueball is close to the other one.

In other words, try to gather the three balls. If you can't, try to leave the first object ball in the center of the table. If that isn't practical, leave all three along a long rail. And if you can't do that, drop the first ball into a corner.

Shots with a Curving Cueball

When a cueball with topspin hits an object ball at an angle the carom path will be curved. Keep in mind that sidespin has practically no effect on the path of the cueball off the object ball—it is topspin and backspin that introduce distortion. How far the cueball travels from the object ball before its path begins to curve depends on how hard you hit it.

Bizarre cueball curves caused by power draws, force follows, and masses are the basis of many sensational exhibition shots. We'll bypass those and present instead a half dozen practical shots that depend on "bending the ball," to use an old San Francisco expression.

Shot 1, Diagram 110, is a cross-table. Note that the red ball is farther from the end rail than the white, which means that the cueball has to travel "uphill" off the first rail to get around the red, then bend forward because of the follow action. A touch of right English is sometimes needed to make the cueball rebound properly off the first rail. The same shot sometimes comes up in the center of the table, where the cueball hits three side rails before scoring.

Shot 2, Diagram 110, is not easy—it's a double-the-rail with the cueball curving around the second ball. Don't shoot too hard or the cueball won't have time to dip into the corner for the third rail. I once saw Boston Shorty make this against Luis Campos with the cueball at the other end of the table.

Shot 3, Diagram 111, demonstrates a common application of follow. Trying to double the rail by going thin off the white is impossible because the angle into the first rail would be too steep. With a full hit, however, the cueball steps sideways before diving forward, hitting the first rail at such a shallow angle that the shot becomes relatively easy.

Shot 4, Diagram 111, is similar to 3, but makes use of draw. The shot

Diagrams 110 and 111: The curving cueball

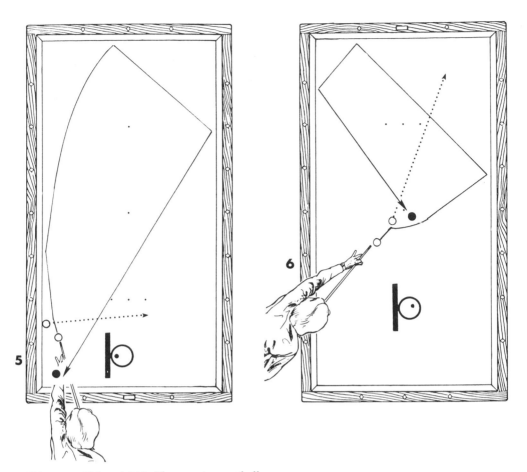

Diagrams 112 and 113: The curving cueball

is so surprising to beginners and laymen that it can be used for showing off.

Shot 5, Diagram 112, is very instructive. The red is big in the corner, but at first sight there seems to be no way to take advantage of it because the white can't be hit thin enough. Or can it? Not with running English. Low draw is needed in order to bend the cueball path as shown. The trick is to hit the white really thin—just barely feather it.

I've seen shots like 6, Diagram 113, passed up by good tournament players in favor of all sorts of goofy wing-dings. It's true that at first sight it looks as though there is no scoring angle off the right side of the white, but don't forget the curve that follow will give it. Practice this one. It comes up all the time and is often overlooked.

Of these six shots, only 2 and 4 are difficult. When faced with them, I would look hard for something better. The others, though, are not bad at all. The student must learn to gobble them up like the cookies they are.

A related subject has to do with what happens when the first object ball is close to a rail or close to a corner. In those cases the cueball hits one or two rails before the follow or draw has a chance to take effect.

The Spin Shot

Pool players seldom have need for tremendous sidespin, but good three-cushion players use it in almost every match. In fact, many pool players don't even know how to apply it, and the question "How do you get so much spin on the ball?" is one billiard players hear all the time. The answer to the question is simple. To make the cueball spin you not only have to hit it off center, you have to hit the object ball full in the face or very nearly so.

I'm talking *English* here—a tremendous amount of English. The shots I'm going to describe require the cueball to travel slowly across the cloth while at the same time spinning furiously. The only way to achieve the effect is to hit the first ball so full that almost all of the speed is removed from the cueball, leaving only the spin. Spin shots can be used to miss kisses, get position, or enlarge the target area on the third ball.

In Diagram 114, consider first the shot with E as the second object ball. If you can send the cueball to point X on the second rail with slow speed and great spin, the shot is almost impossible to miss because of the angle the cueball will take off the third rail. In planning the shot in your head, ignore the first rail and choose instead a likely spot on the second rail, keeping in mind how slowly the cueball will be traveling and how fast it will be spinning as compared to a cueball with normal running English. Be sure to hit it hard enough so the cueball is still spinning when it reaches the third rail, and keep in mind too that it is almost impossible to miss the shot "short."

If the second object ball is at F instead of E, a much different contact point is needed on the second rail, labeled Y in the diagram. For second-object-ball position G, the cueball would have to hit the second rail at or

Diagram 114. Spin shots

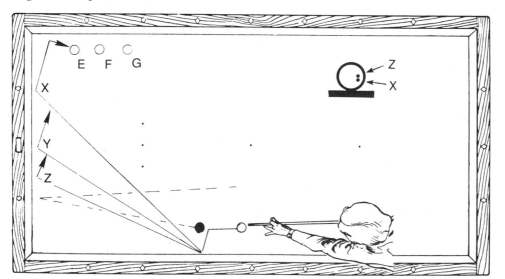

near point Z. The dashed line shows the approximate path of the first object ball. Note that the hit is almost full. (A completely full hit with English only and no follow or draw would leave the cueball spinning in place.) The hit on the first ball in the three cases can be identical, with the path of the cueball to the second rail determined only by the precise nature of the English. The enlarged cueball shows that a slightly below-center hit will draw the cueball to point X, while a slightly above-center hit will send the cueball to point Z.

A certain touch is required, and if you've never tried the shot you almost certainly will need a demonstration by a good player before you can get the hang of it. Once you can send the cueball to any desired spot on the second rail, the three diagrammed shots become high-percentage chances.

At the left of Diagram 115 is a short-angle shot that could be made with no English or slight running English, but the third rail would have to be contacted with great precision. A spin shot greatly improves the chance of scoring. An authoritative stroke rather than precision is called for. The cueball in the given position must go slightly "uphill" into the first rail; a perpendicular path into the first rail would cause the cueball to hit the second rail too far from the red ball.

At the right of Diagram 115 is a shot I saw Ceulemans make. The red ball was almost frozen, which meant that the target on the third rail was extremely small. A force follow with spin, as drawn, sent the cueball into the third rail slowly while spinning at high speed, providing a target a couple of inches wide. A slippery new cloth is best for this kind of action because the spin doesn't die out as quickly.

The shot in Diagram 116 I learned from the late Jimmy Lee of San

Diagram 115. Spin shots

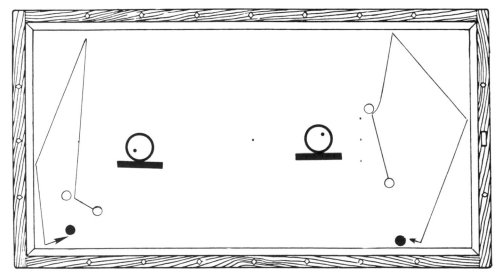

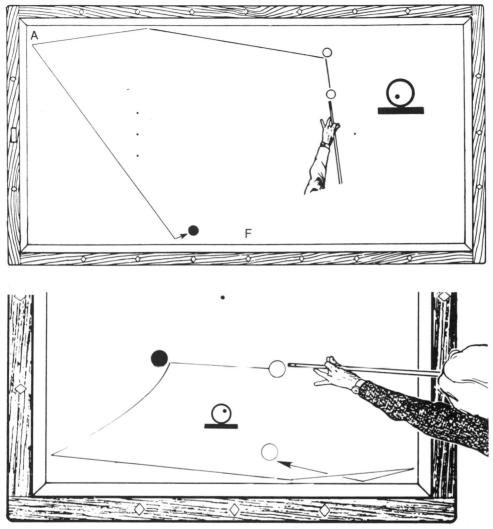

Diagrams 116 and 117: Spin shots

Francisco. As a spin shot it is almost a cinch. If you can send the cueball toward the corner slowly with maximum spin, it will take an angle off the second rail that will bring it to a point near the third diamond on the third rail. The first object ball, provided it is within six inches or so of the first rail, can be almost anywhere along the length of the table. It is possible to reach point F, opposite the fourth diamond on the third rail, if you can send the cueball deep into the corner at A. (See also Diagram 84.)

The through-the-hole double-the-rail pattern drawn in Diagram 117 is not normally called a spin shot, but it has two characteristics after the cueball leaves the first rail—slow speed and tremendous spin. It is stroked as a force follow with high right-hand English. The speed on the cueball is killed not by the full hit but by the negative angle of approach into the first rail. The action is beautiful because the cueball speeds up after hitting the fourth rail.

I cry real tears for players forced to play on tables with cheap, coarse cloth that takes away many spin-shot options. If your proprietor is too cheap to provide imported cloth, I urge you to take up a collection and buy it yourself. Go to a billiard supply store and ask for Simonis (Belgium) or Granito (Spain). To a much greater degree than pool, the pleasure to be derived from three cushion is dependent upon the quality of the equipment. If the rubber on your table is dead and the cloth is cheap or worn out, you might as well go bowling.

The Jump Shot

The jump shot in pool has become a popular weapon among today's top players in recent years. Opportunities for jump shots also come up in three-cushion billiards, but not nearly as often. Billiard jump shots are more often used in exhibitions than in games—still, there are a few positions where they are practical, especially for the aggressive player.

Years ago, a standard shot among three-cushion professionals involved sending the first object ball off the table to eliminate a kiss. That stratagem was banned by the international ruling body a decade or two ago, perhaps at the request of room owners and clubs, for the jump shot is admittedly hard on equipment. The way I understand the rules now, jump shots are legal provided no ball touches the wooden part of the rail; a ball riding along the top of the cushion before falling back onto the table is okay.

I discuss jump shots here with some uneasiness. What proprietor in his right mind would let you practice them? The following, therefore, is aimed only at those who can get to a billiard table secretly.

In executing jump shots, the cue must be elevated. How high depends on how high you want the cueball to rise (45 degrees is about the limit; more than that and it is too hard to aim and stroke). Speed also varies with the amount of jump needed, but most jump shots must be hit with considerable authority. You can apply right and left English and backspin to the cueball on a jump shot, but forget about topspin because the tip will interfere with the ball's effort to leave the cloth.

The jump shot in Diagram 118 may well be the best choice under the circumstances. There are several other shots to consider, but they can be made tougher with a slight change in the placement of the balls. Shooting down on the cueball with enough power to make it jump over the red gives you a good chance of scoring. Some left English is needed in the given position, and the resulting massé effect is shown by the curve in the cueball's path on its way to the first rail. The shot is also possible when the balls are a few inches to the right, in which case the cueball sometimes rides the top of the cushion for a few feet.

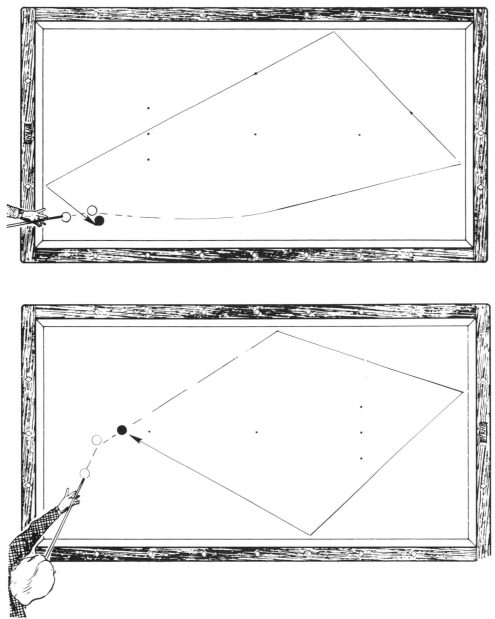

Diagrams 118 and 119: Jump shots

The shot in Diagram 119 is eminently practical. In fact, at one Western Regional Tournament in North Hollywood, I was playing at the table next to Al Gilbert when he made the shot in a game against John Teerink of Seattle. Gilbert had to jump the entire red ball. The shot is a little easier, of course, when you only have to jump over the edge of a ball.

The shot in Diagram 120 is by no means as hard as it looks. The idea is to shoot with an elevated cue into a ball frozen to a rail and then jump back over the second ball, going around the table, as shown, to score. I don't mean to imply that it is *easy*, which is why I have rolled up my sleeve in

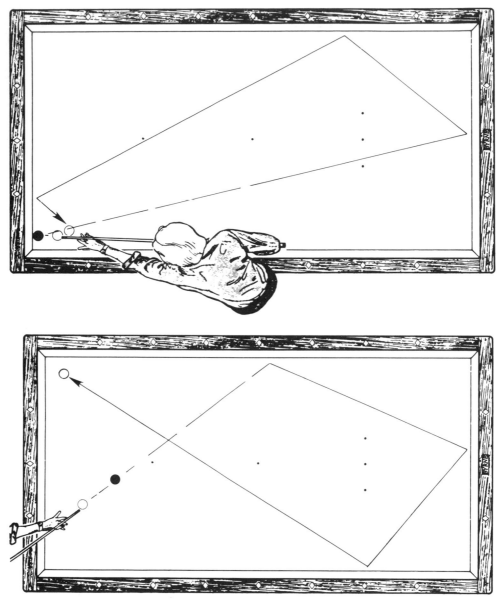

Diagrams 120 and 121: Jump shots

the drawing, but once a good player gets the hang of it he may be able to make it one time in three. It helps to use a bit of draw as well as left English on the cueball, otherwise the cueball will slow up on its way to the other end of the table.

In Diagram 121, a tempting shot is a force follow through the red. Unfortunately, there is a good chance that the red ball will take the same path intended for the cueball and will kiss the second ball out of the way before the cueball arrives. One solution that I discovered on my own is a jump shot that enables the cueball to *almost* clear the red ball. The cueball hits the top part of the red as it passes over it and continues around the

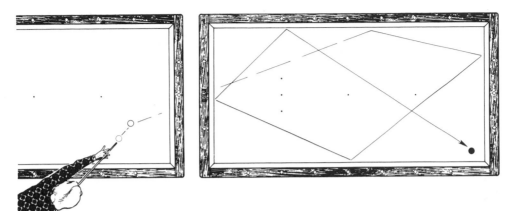

Diagram 122. Jump shots

table in front of the red. The basic idea goes back at least to the early years of the last century. Minguad, who is credited with inventing the leather tip and was the world's first professional exhibition player, had a shot on a pocket table in which the object ball and the cueball were lined up straight into the corner pocket. He made the cueball go into the pocket first, followed by the object ball, by using a jump shot that doesn't quite clear the object ball.

Jumping the cueball from one table to another, as in Diagram 122, is another idea that goes back a couple of hundred years. In billiards, the trick shooter usually tries to make a three-rail bank on the second table, but since you have to use a lot of power to send the ball across the gap between tables (pushed together here to save space), you might as well try for a five-railer and a standing ovation.

This only scratches the surface of the subject (as well as the surface of the balls). There are more in *Byrne's Treasury of Trick Shots*, where 23 jump shots are diagrammed—15 for pool and 8 for billiards.

The Cross-table Shot

Much of three-cushion billiards is a matter of adapting several dozen basic patterns to specific ball positions. One frequently occurring pattern is the cross-table shot. In this section we'll look at a few positions in which the point is scored without making use of the end rails.

Don't pay too much attention to the exact placements of the balls— the idea of the shot is the important thing. First learn to recognize the shot, then through practice and experience become familiar with how the cueball behaves with various amounts of speed and English.

In the shot given in Diagram 123, the first object ball must be struck fairly full to drive it out of the way of a kiss off the first rail and to enable the cueball to approach the second rail at an angle. If the cueball hits the

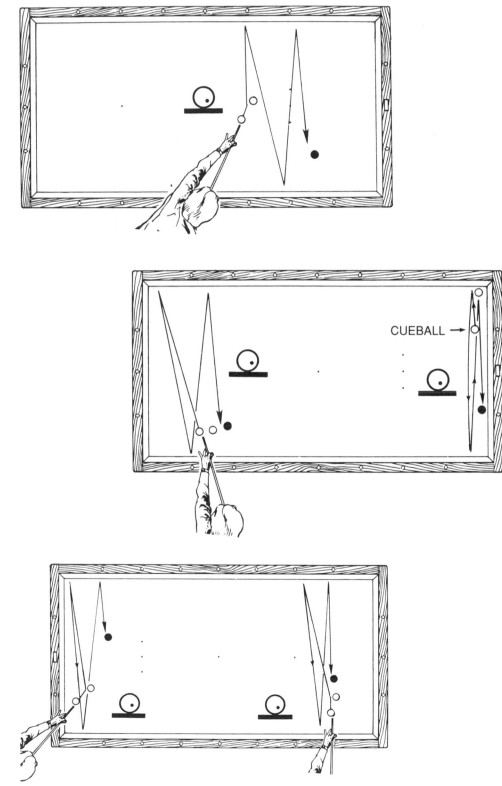

CUEBALL →

second rail too close to the perpendicular it will tend not to continue "walking" down the table—residual English, in fact, might make it "back up" and draw farther away from the red ball the second time across. To make the cueball zigzag down the table in the proper "W" pattern, it usually helps to use low English as well as side and to *elevate the cue a little*. The shot as diagrammed brings out an important point in positions of this type—the red ball is "big" even though it is a foot away from the nearest rail. If the cueball misses it off the third rail it may catch it off the fourth or even the fifth. That's why cross-table shots have a higher percentage of scoring than they sometimes first appear.

The need for establishing the proper angle into the second rail is obvious on the left side of Diagram 124. Unless the first rail is approached at a negative or backward angle there is no scoring path. I show the cueball hitting the first rail a full diamond below its origin on the near rail, which is about the limit on most tables. The shot at the right of the diagram is not easy, but all other options are practically impossible. Strike the first ball extremely thin with low right and with firm speed. The nice thing about the shot is that it works no matter where the red ball is along the rail. Sometimes the cueball picks up the end rail.

The shot at the left in Diagram 125 is similar to Diagram 123 but shifted close to the left end. When I saw Raymond Ceulemans try the shot in the 1974 world tournament, I asked him after the game why he didn't try a short angle. His answer was that in the cross-table the red ball was huge. Miss it off the third rail and you might make it off the fourth. The shot at the right of the diagram is quite similar but is almost always overlooked if the red ball is farther from the end rail than the white ball. It would be easier if it weren't, but it is still possible.

The shot at the left in Diagram 126, which was shown to me by the

Diagram 126. Cross-table shots

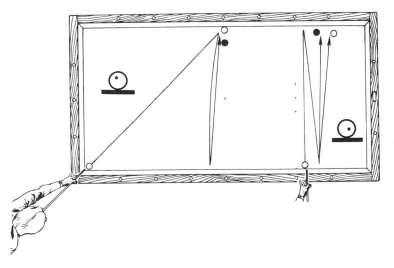

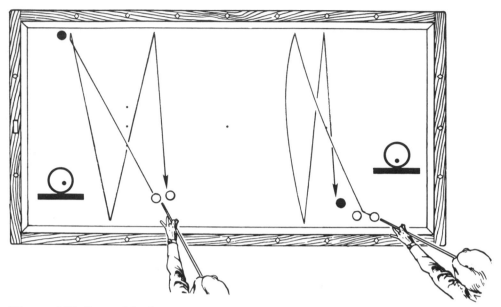

Diagram 127. Cross-table shots

late Danny McGoorty, is presented as a challenge, a test of skill. Hit the first ball fairly thin and not too hard. Practice it at first without freezing the cueball in the corner.

When faced with the shot at the right in Diagram 126, most players would probably try a three-rail natural bank around the table, but with the balls as shown a two-way cross-table is better. Note that the cueball can hit either object ball first. Compare this to shots 182 and 183 in *Byrne's Standard Book*. See also shot 58 in Willie Hoppe's *Billiards As It Should Be Played*.

American players almost never think of the "uphill" cross-table given at the left of Diagram 127. I've seen Ceulemans try it and make it from positions even more difficult than this. It's actually a fairly easy shot when the cueball is within a foot or two of the first ball.

The shot at the right of Diagram 127 may not seem practical, but it is. Use straight draw—no English. Believe it or not, the shot can be made even if the red ball is two more diamonds to the left.

Drop-ins and Holdups

The two shots in Diagram 128 illustrate a subtlety that was shown to me many years ago by Rene Vingerhoedt of Belgium, who was world champion just before Ceulemans. A typical position is shown at the left of Diagram 128. The surest way to handle it is to hit the first ball half full, using just enough left English to bring the cueball back across the table along the

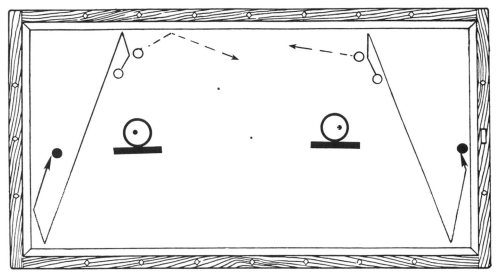

Diagram 128. Drop-ins and holdups

correct scoring path. After leaving the first rail, the cueball should have no English. The dashed line indicates roughly how much white ball to hit.

The position at the right of the diagram is identical with the exception of the red ball, which is on the rail. If you use the same technique as before, the third target is very small. Instead, hit less of the object ball and bring the cueball back across the table with some English. Now when it hits the second rail, the reverse or "hold up" English will tend to keep it more parallel with the end rail, enlarging the target.

A note about safety play in shots like this. If you shoot softly in order to die near the red, you will leave your opponent's cueball at the other end of the table, but you will also increase the chances of leaving yourself tough if you should score. (Scoring when you are playing safe is called shooting through your own safety.) It's better to use enough speed to make the white ball bounce off the far end rail a distance of two or three diamonds. That way you won't have so much green to cross if you score and the leave dictates going off the white on the next shot.

If the red ball is past the center of the table, as at the left of Diagram 129, an option that must be considered in the so-called twice-across shot. The third rail target is much bigger than it is in the previous pattern. It seems obvious as drawn, but for some reason the pattern is often overlooked when the balls are moved several feet toward the center of the table.

At the right of Diagram 129, is a spin shot. If the first ball is hit fairly full, the cueball will return across the table spinning like a top. When the "hole" between the red and the end rail is small it is, of course, best to follow the dashed line; when the hole is large, the solid line path must be considered. An advantage of the solid line path is that reverse English on the second and third rails kills the speed of the cueball, leaving it far from the other cueball if you miss.

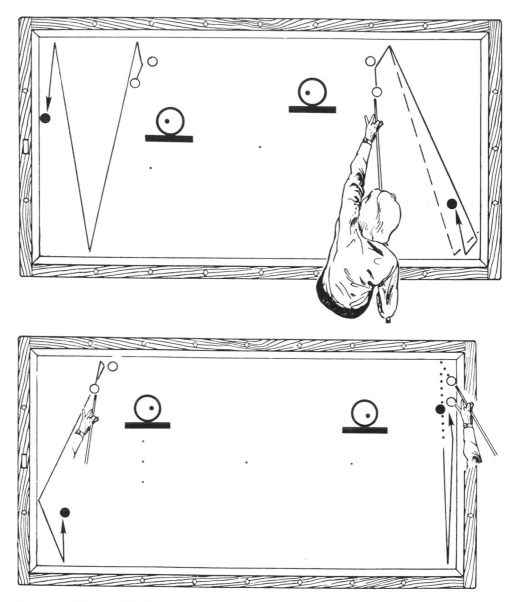

Diagrams 129 and 130: Drop-ins and holdups

When the first ball is close to the rail you have another option, and that is hitting the rail first as shown at the left of Diagram 130. From the angle given, I would find it much easier to predict the path of the cueball with a rail-first hit.

The last shot, at the right of Diagram 130, is for the advanced player and is a creation of San Francisco's Bud Harris. The two white balls are frozen to the rail. Bud's idea is to elevate the cue and shoot into the side rail so that the cueball jumps over the red, as indicated by the dotted line. Right English is used to bring the cueball across the table at the proper angle.

While the shot is fancy enough to be used as a trick shot, it is perfectly practical under game conditions and is not as hard as it looks.

The thinking behind the six shots described here is also applicable to positions in which the cueball travels the length rather than the width of the table.

Diamond Systems

You don't need to know any of the diamond systems in three-cushion billiards to be world champion. Welker Cochran and Willie Hoppe, two of the greatest players of all time, did not use arithmetic in their games, relying solely on judgment and experience. And Raymond Ceulemans claims to have won his first three world championships without familiarity with system play.

Systems help, but they aren't essential and they certainly aren't infallible. I can't help wondering about the identity of the comedian who claims in recent editions of the BCA rule book that the system "takes all the guesswork out of three cushion billiards." Most top players today, though, especially the Americans and Japanese, make use of several types of systems to assist them in picking the right spot to aim for on the first rail. The other two major variables on every shot, speed and spin, remain a matter of "touch." Some systems are designed to determine the amount of spin, measured in "tips" from the center of the cueball.

What follows is an introduction to the most widely used system, "the corner five," a look at two "distant point" systems, and remarks that may help beginners and intermediate players put together what they already know so that they can become practical tools and not just interesting intellectual exercises. Remember, the description here is far from complete and refers to just three systems. There are scores of others.

The corner five system involves three sets of numbers, one for the origin of the cueball, one for the first rail, and one for the third rail. The numbers are assigned to the table as shown in Diagrams 131 and 132. The cueball origin is determined by noting where the cue crosses the rail. In the first diagram, the cueball aimed by the player is originating, in effect, from the corner (ignore the arrow for the moment). The cueball number for the shot diagrammed, therefore, is 5.0. Since the cueball is aimed at first rail number 3.0, it will go into third rail number 2.0 because the difference between 5.0 and 3.0 is 2.0. That relationship between the three sets of numbers is the basis of the system.

Note that when aiming the cueball you direct it through the rubber to the desired diamond on the wooden part of the rail. Don't aim at a point on

Diagrams 131, 132, and 133: The diamond systems

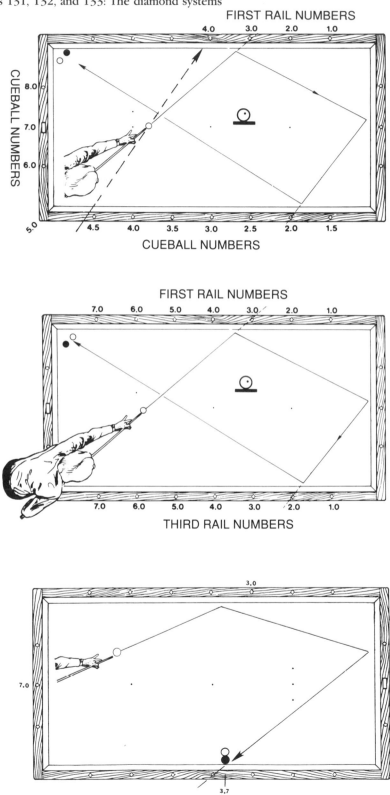

FIRST RAIL NUMBERS

4.0   3.0   2.0   1.0

CUEBALL NUMBERS

8.0
7.0
6.0
5.0

4.5   4.0   3.5   3.0   2.5   2.0   1.5

CUEBALL NUMBERS

FIRST RAIL NUMBERS

7.0   6.0   5.0   4.0   3.0   2.0   1.0

7.0   6.0   5.0   4.0   3.0   2.0   1.0

THIRD RAIL NUMBERS

3.0

7.0

3.7

the nose of the rubber opposite the diamond. Also, on most tables, the cueball travels toward the third rail along a line leading toward the calculated third rail diamond and not at the point on the rubber opposite it.

Many system shots are missed because the third rail target is improperly chosen. Diagram 133 shows that the cueball must approach 4.0 on the third rail to score the point, even though the balls are opposite 3.7.

I know several good players of long experience who don't use the diamond system because they have never been clearly told that the cueball has no "number" or "origin" until it has been aimed somewhere. In diagram 131, if the cueball is aimed at 3.0 on the first rail, as the player is doing, then by tracing the line of the cue backward it can be seen that, in effect, the cueball is originating from the corner, which is called 5.0. However, if the cueball is aimed at 4.0 on the first rail, as indicated by the arrow, then the cueball is, in effect, starting from 4.6. Finding the right place to aim on the first rail in order to reach a predetermined spot on the third rail is a matter of trial and error as the player tries to find two numbers whose difference equals the third rail number. Unless the cueball is on the rail to start with, every new point on the first rail it is aimed at results in a new effective starting point.

The system described here is quite accurate in reaching points on the third rail, although from some extreme cueball origins, like 8.0 and 2.0, substantial adjustments must be made. The angle the cueball takes off the third rail depends on where the cueball started from. The system charts in Willie Hoppe's *Billiards As It Should Be Played* are almost useless because they show the cueball connecting from the second diamond on the third rail to the diagonally opposite corner no matter where the cueball begins. Diagram 134 shows how the cueball "tracks" shift between the third and

Diagram 134. The diamond systems

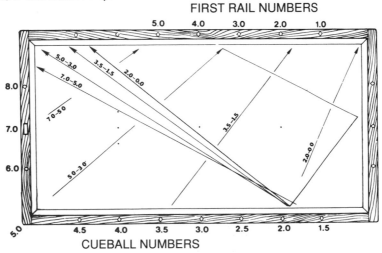

fourth rails as the cueball origin changes. These shifts must be understood and compensated for.

The method I like best for coping with track shifts is described in detail in *Byrne's Standard Book* (as are the other points raised here) and involves noting how far from the 5.0 corner the cueball origin is and expressing that distance as a percentage of the whole rail. For example, say you want to bank the cueball three rails into the corner as in Diagram 131 but you are shooting out of cueball number 4.0 instead of 5.0. If you were shooting out of 5.0, you would know that 2.0 on the third rail connects with the corner. (Returns such as this should be memorized from the start.) To reach 2.0 on the third rail from cueball number 4.0 suggests a first rail number of 2.0, but an allowance must be made because the cueball is not coming from the "natural" corner number 5.0. An allowance of a quarter diamond is made on the first rail because cueball number 4.0 is a quarter of the way down the rail from the corner. Therefore, you aim the cueball at 1.75 instead of 2.0 on the first rail.

Points to remember:

1. Tables differ. Even the same table will differ in its angles depending on which direction the cueball is shot. You must adapt the system to fit the table.
2. Aim through to the diamond on the first rail, not opposite it.
3. Assume that the cueball will travel through the rail to the desired third rail point, not opposite it.
4. Use running English and firm speed. To find out how much English, repeat the shot in Diagram 131 until you can put the cueball in the corner off the third rail.
5. The angle off the third rail depends on where the cueball starts from.
6. The further you get from cueball number 5.0, the more important are judgment and touch.
7. Unless you have a method of making allowances, the corner five system is not a practical tool.
8. The first step in planning a system shot is to estimate the third rail number. The next step is to aim the cueball at various points on the first rail until you find a first rail number that differs by the desired amount from the cueball origin. The difference must be equal to the third rail number.
9. The diamond system does not take all the guesswork out of three-cushion billiards.

Systems are a big help on many shots, not just bank shots, and are always useful backup for judgment.

Not all systems involve adding and subtracting fractions or decimals. There are, for example, the so-called "spot-on-the-wall" systems, which I prefer to call "distant point" because the wall might not be the right distance away. I'll briefly describe an end-rail system shown to me by Don Brink of Raytown, Mo., and a reverse English system shown to me by Jim Friel of the Denver Athletic Club.

The distant point can be any easy-to-see target—a chair leg, an ashtray, a spectator's foot, a post, a design on a rug . . . or a spot on the wall. The idea is that once the appropriate distant point is selected for a certain arrangement of object balls, the cueball is aimed toward it. It doesn't make any difference where the cueball is.

There seems to be no agreement on how far away from the table the aiming point should be. I find that between ten and twelve feet is about right for the system described here: A difference of about a foot or two changes the cueball's path by only the slightest amount.

In Diagram 135 the cueball is frozen on the rail near the second diamond, as shown. You have decided to try the shot as shown in Diagram 136—end-rail first. Here's how you find a distant point to use as an aiming target. Estimate the point of the third rail you think you have to hit to score the billiard. To facilitate the explanation, I'll call that point a. Note the distance from a to the corner (line a–b) and mentally mark off the same distance at the diagonally opposite corner (d–c). Keeping one eye on point c, walk to corner E and sight through it to point c and extend the line of sight to a distant point, here marked P. (To save space in the diagram, P is closer to the table than it should be.) Now that you have established the location of P, all you have to do is aim the cueball at it with running English, as shown in Diagram 136. The cueball can be anywhere above the dotted line. You'll have to try it a few times to get the feel of how much English to use. You won't make the shot every time, but at least you'll look good missing.

Before playing a game on any table, it pays to bank the cueball around in several different patterns, keeping your eyes open. One bank I always try is the reverse English out of the corner, given in Diagram 137. Put the cueball on a line between corner E and the center of the long rail, here marked a, and shoot softly with maximum reverse English (see inset). On most tables the cueball will hit the third rail near the point marked c. If you change the line of aim and hit a third of a diamond to the right, point b, the cueball hits the third rail a diamond farther from the corner, at point d.

If a shot comes up during the game in which the cueball must be made to come off point c on the third rail, and if the cueball is not originating from corner E, then all you have to do is aim at P, which is the distant point found by projecting the line of aim you would use if the cueball *was* in the corner. Similarly, if d is where you want to hit on the third rail, first stand at E, project a line to b on the first rail, extend the line ten or twelve feet to Q, and aim the cueball at that. Remember, use heavy reverse English and slow speed.

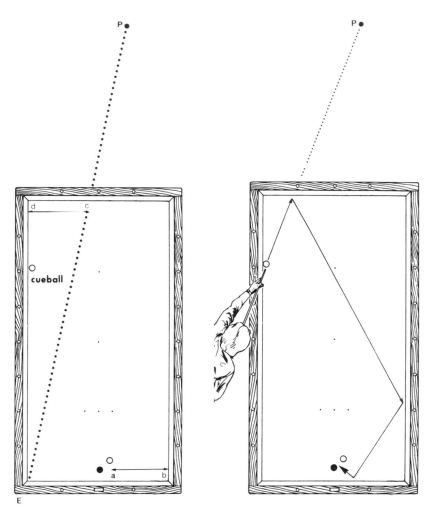

Diagrams 135 and 136: The diamond systems

Now you have a way of mapping out the beautiful ball-first shot given in Diagram 138 and finding out where the cueball must hit on the first rail. First, estimate where on the third rail the cueball must hit to score the point, keeping in mind that the cueball will have extra spin since it will be coming off the ball. Next stand at corner A and pick the point on the first rail you'd have to hit if the cueball was in that corner. In this case the point is a little to the right of the center of the long rail—an educated guess based on the practice banks you took before the game started. Project the direction of aim (long dotted line) beyond the first rail to a distant point (not shown in the diagram). Walk to point B and, by sighting along the edge of the first object ball, find a line that leads to the distant point. Where that line crosses the first rail is the point the cueball has to hit when it comes off the object ball with reverse English. Hitting the first ball a little too full won't hurt because then the cueball will arrive at the third rail with less speed and more spin, which makes the red ball large.

Diagrams 137 and 138: The diamond systems

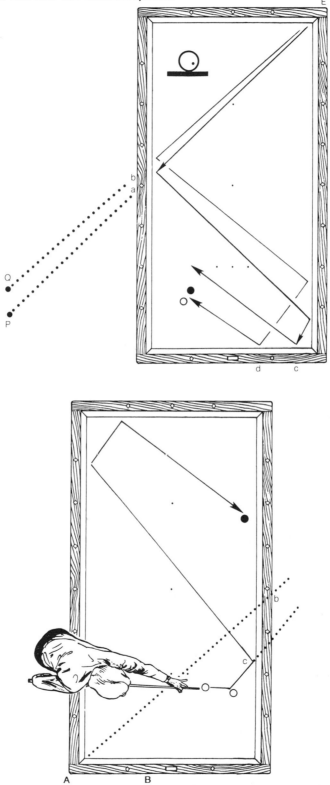

The Stroke Shots of Artistic Billiards

What American billiard players call exhibition shots, fancy shots, or skill shots are called artistic or fantasy billiards in the rest of the world. So fond are the Europeans of the big-stroke follow, draw, jump, and massé shots that for 40 years they've been holding tournaments in them. The organization that sponsors them is called the Commission Internationale de Billard Artisique (CIBA).

This typical CIBA tournament consists of 76 difficult shots set up the same way for each contestant, although *precise* ball placement is not as crucial for most of the shots as it is for many pool table trick shots. "Trick shots" is certainly not the right term to use when talking about artistic billiards. There is nothing tricky about them. Most of them are just plain monsters that require not only an understanding of a specialized body of knowledge but a King Kong stroke.

Each player in the tournament is given three tries to make each shot in the program, and success gives the player a number of points that changes with the difficulty of the shot. Making an easy one might net as few as four points, the hardest one as many as eleven. The winner of the world tournament (who will probably be from Spain or Belgium) will score on about half of the shots. Because the shots are weighted for scoring purposes, the winning total will usually be between 250 and 300.

Until recently, it was almost impossible to find out how to spot the balls for the various shots. The only diagrams were in tournament programs and were too small to be very useful. The situation has now been corrected. Bob Jewett, the former national intercollegiate pool champion, has dug out the necessary information, drawn with engineering precision the 76 shots on 8½-by-11-inch graph paper—drawings that include the sometimes bizarre path the cueball must take to score—described the system used to spot the balls for each shot, and provided a few words of background, all of which is contained in an 88-page photocopied booklet. (For a copy, send $12 to Billiard Library, 1570 Seabright Ave., Long Beach, Calif. 90813.)

The availability of the Jewett monograph raises the possibility that the United States can begin participating in the world artistic billiard tournament. At least now American players know what the shots are and can practice them. (Provided they have their own tables or know lenient proprietors. A good time to work on massé shots is the day before the cloth is to be changed.) Interest is growing in staging an American tournament, the winner of which would advance to the world.

Turning to the diagrammed shots, Diagram 139 is a rail-first follow, reversing off the third rail, and would not be too bad a choice in a game of three cushion, especially if the red ball were frozen. This is a fairly easy shot compared to the others and is worth only five points in competition.

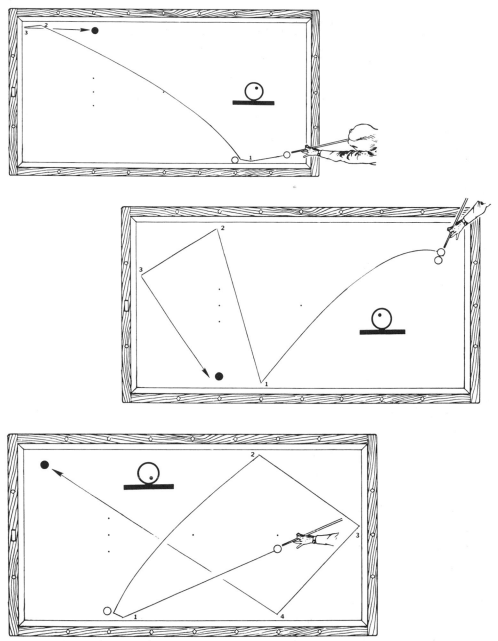

Diagrams 139, 140, and 141: Stroke shots

In Diagram 140 the cueball is not quite frozen to the object ball. The shot is a force-follow reverse and is rated at eight points. Elevate the cue about 20 degrees.

You think you have a good stroke? Then try the rail first around-the-table draw given in Diagram 141. Make it once in three tries and you get nine points.

Many players might argue that the cross-table draw shot in Diagram 142 is impossible. To the master players who specialize in this sort of thing

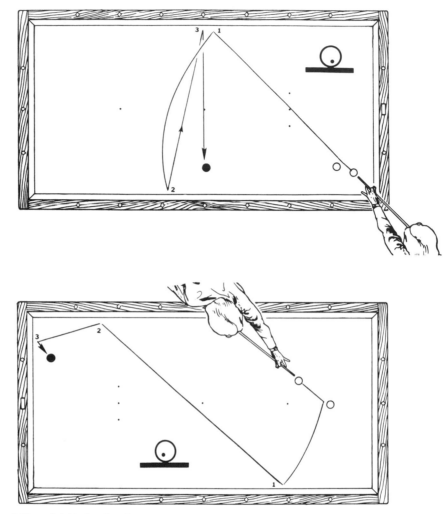

Diagrams 142 and 143: Stroke shots

it is not only possible, it is not even particularly difficult. Make it in artistic competition and you get only six points.

Diagram 143 is a reverse English draw that is considered hard enough to be worth eight points.

Diagram 144 is the dreaded "big massé." To score, the cueball must contact the first rail to left of the point marked X. This is an impressive shot to see—the cueball gains speed rapidly between the first and second rails. Eight points. The cue is held close to vertical.

A jump draw is given in Diagram 145. Elevate the cue about 45 degrees and use low right. The cueball knocks the white out without disturbing the red, jumps over the red, then curves back as shown. It is not necessary to hit three rails in this one, and it is considered so easy by the experts that they give themselves only six points when they make it once in three tries.

Diagram 146 is worth ten points. (In competition the cueball is placed

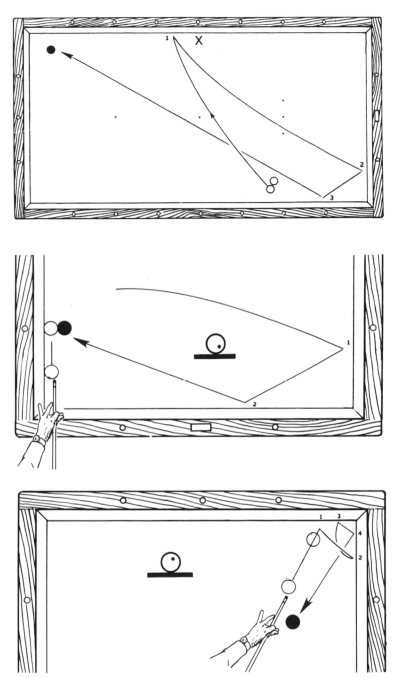

Diagrams 144, 145, and 146: Stroke shots

about a foot farther away from the first object ball.) If a really gross amount of follow is imparted to the cueball, it will continue fighting its way into the corner until five or even six rails are contacted.

Wondering what an eleven looks like? Shoot Diagram 141 as a straight draw off the white; that is, without the rail first. That's an eleven.

Thirty-seven Shots from Master Play

One of my hobbies is attending three-cushion billiard tournaments and making diagrams of unusual or instructive shots. The shots in Diagrams 147–152 are from a 1979 tournament held at California Billiards in San Jose, Calif.

The shot in Diagram 147 was pulled off by Bud Harris of San Francisco. A four-railer off the red was too tough because it would have been necessary to shoot over a ball. Instead, Harris played two rails first as diagrammed, feathering the white, then picking up three more rails before striking the red. The applause he received was well deserved. Later Harris was faced with the difficult position in Diagram 148. His solution to the problem was to "manufacture" an angle with the use of draw, making the cueball curve after leaving the first rail. Note slight holdup English.

The $75 prize for high run out of the money was shared by Nabih Yousri and myself for our strings of nine. One of the shots I made in my run

Diagrams 147 and 148: Shots from master play

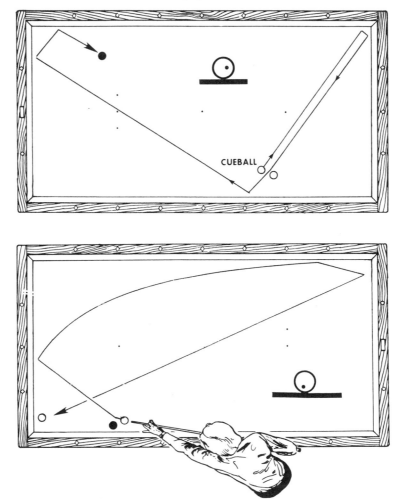

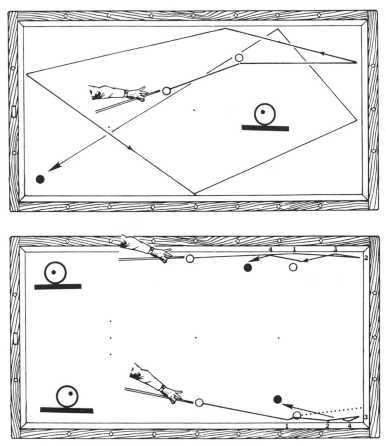

Diagrams 149 and 150: Shots from master play

was the six-railer in Diagram 149, which is not particularly remarkable on fast Granito cloth. On a slow table it is essential to hit the first ball thin so that not much speed is transferred to the first object ball.

The shot at the top of Diagram 150, which I call a through-the-hole backup ticky, was made by Carlos Hallon. Again, this shot is not difficult when the balls are placed as shown. The trick is to think of it. Little speed is needed. Use this pattern when it is not possible to hit the end rail first. (For newcomers to the game who are unable to catch the idea of this shot because of the small scale of the diagram, the cueball hits three rails first, then hits the white ball, a fourth rail, and finally the red ball.)

Also in Diagram 150 is champion Al Gilbert's out shot against fourth-place finisher Don Brink of Kansas City. It is a follow ticky reverse. The white ball is about a finger-width away from the rail. The cueball contacts the first rail farther away from the first object ball than it would on an ordinary ticky so that it *follows through* the ball instead of going immediately back to the rail. The reverse follow made the cueball double the rail after hitting the first ball. The same idea can be used with running English when it is not necessary to come back to the long rail. Many players pass up tickys in which the first ball is less than a ball-width away from the rail and the red is close to the corner because they think there is no way to keep the cueball close to the rail. It can be done with the following idea. When hit right the first ball does not diverge very much from the long rail, as indicated by the dotted line. This valuable shot is impossible to describe clearly in words. The action sometimes occurs by accident when the player is trying to go rail-first off the outside of the ball for a cross-table pattern. If the cueball has some speed, the rubber is depressed and the cueball goes through a hole that doesn't seem large enough, staying close to the long rail all the way to the corner.

An enjoyable feature of billiard tournaments is the postmortem sessions in which the players demonstrate shots they made or missed in their games or set up memorable shots from yesteryear. Nabih Yousri set up the shot in Diagram 151, which was his out shot in a tournament game in Egypt 15 years earlier. It is a four-rail first reverse bank, with a firm stroke and high English to lengthen the angle off the first rail.

The shot in Diagram 152 is a gem Yousri made during the San Jose tournament.

Diagrams 151 and 152: Shots from master play

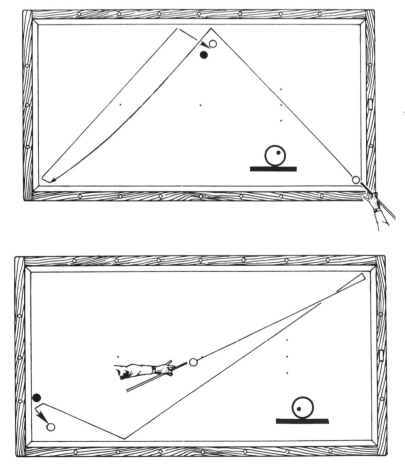

Every top three-cushion player has a good imagination and a good memory. When they find the balls in an unusual position, they can either make up a shot to suit their circumstances, relying on their knowledge of how balls behave with various speeds and spins, or they trust their memory of how somebody else handled the shot months or even years earlier. Experience won't help if you can't remember what you've learned.

Some patterns are applicable only once every 5,000 shots or so, but if you recognize them when you see them and if you can recall, even vaguely, what happened last time you tried a certain rare shot, you've got an edge on the player whose mind isn't as retentive.

In Diagrams 153–158 are seven shots that may not strike you as practical at first sight. The serious student, though, will try them a few times and file them away where he can get at them on special occasions. A seldom-used special tool might be just what you need to get out of a tight spot.

The shot in Diagram 153 goes back over 100 years and is said to have been a special favorite of the great Alfredo DeOro. It's a beautiful idea and not as hard as it looks. Often overlooked, even by expert players.

Faced with the position in Diagram 154, most players would probably

Diagrams 153 and 154: Shots from master play

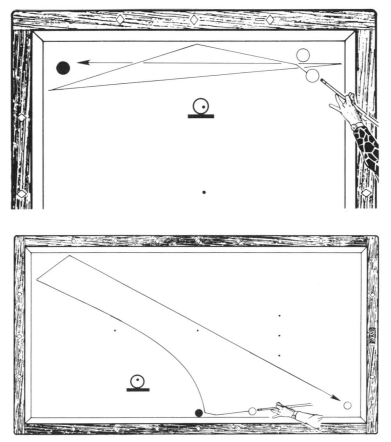

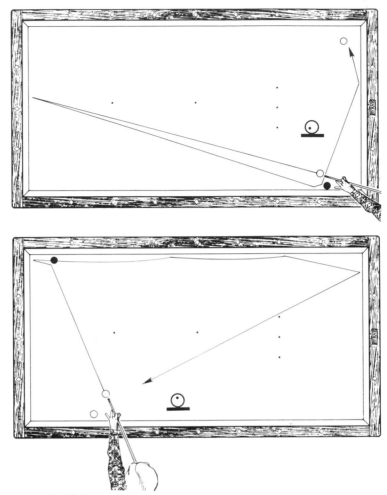

Diagrams 155 and 156: Shots from master play

go off the outside of the red and hope to get a third rail near the white. Others might try a rail shot first with a thin hit on the red. Best is to hit the rail first and the red *full*, as drawn. Use high follow and no more than a trace of running English. This shot is feasible only if the cueball is within a half-inch or so of the rail.

The shot in Diagram 155 is difficult, but is there anything easier? Five rails off the red would be a possibility if you could reach it. The creative solution in the diagram appears in an old book by Kinrey Matsuyama. Without the manufactured angle of approach to the red ball there is no chance at all.

Consider the pattern in Diagram 156. Shoot hard and use plenty of follow and you'll be surprised at how consistently the cueball seeks out the lower left-hand area of the table. Getting the upper long rail twice is not essential.

In Diagram 157 the idea in both shots is to hit the rail first with running

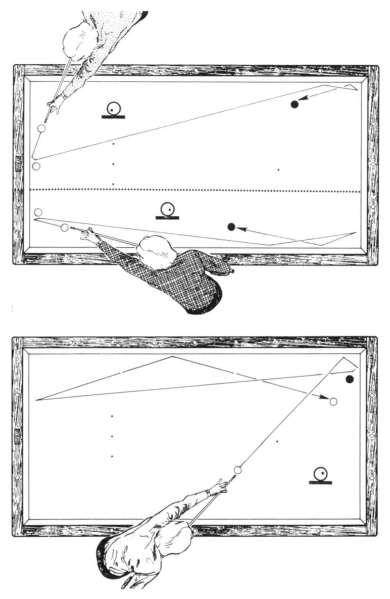

Diagrams 157 and 158: Shots from master play

English, go through the hole formed by the red and the rail, and double the rail before scoring.

The unusual concept in Diagram 158 is better than it seems at first sight because if the cueball comes off the red even approximately right there are many scoring paths to the white.

The next five shots are from tournaments in Krefeld, West Germany, and Metz, France, which I attended in 1984. Four are by the great Raymond Ceulemans of Belgium.

Consider the shots in Diagrams 159 and 160. I was sitting within ten feet of the table when Ceulemans made them and in neither case did I know what he was trying to do until he pulled the trigger. I doubt if any American player would have thought of them, much less made them, because they require massé strokes that aren't in the arsenals of players who restrict themselves to three cushion.

In Diagram 159 there are a couple of banks that could be tried, but Ceulemans hardly considered them. Owner of one of the world's most secure massé strokes, he executed the shot as shown with little trouble, shooting softly.

The shot in Diagram 160 had everybody puzzled while he was aiming it. Nobody had any idea what he had in mind. I wasn't able to jump out of the bleachers and peer over his shoulder, but I believe I have the position drawn correctly. He stood at A *and with his cue almost vertical* sent the cueball to the corner at D with no sidespin, only follow. The cueball stayed flat and came straight across the table to score. (I have omitted the player from the diagram to avoid covering up the shot.) Enough of the red ball was hit so that it moved about a foot and almost kissed the cueball out at R. Again, a fairly soft stroke was used. The crosshairs and the dot on the cueball are intended to show that the cueball was struck exactly on the line of aim, not off to one side, which would impart curve and unwanted running English.

Diagram 159. Shots from master play

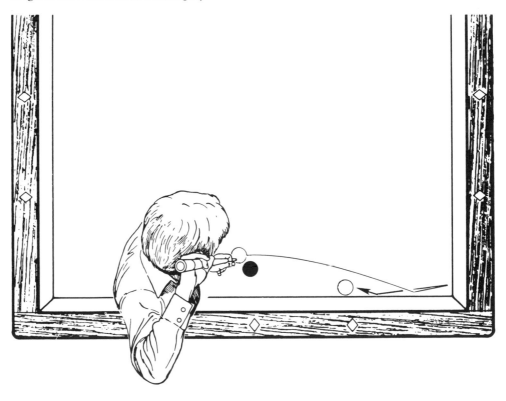

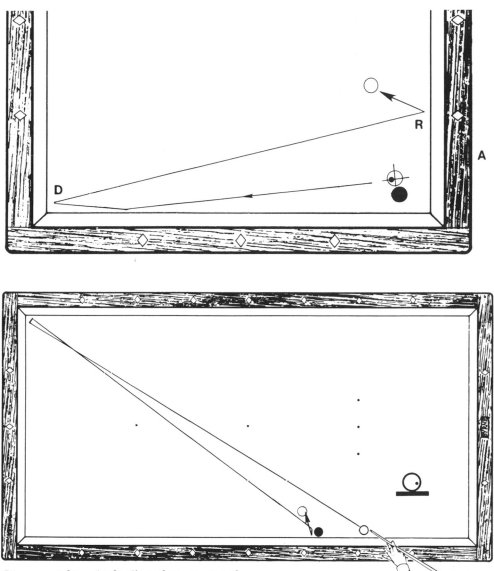

Diagrams 160 and 161: Shots from master play

Only a great master would know, facing this shot in a game, that the cueball could be made to come dead out of the corner.

Ceulemans is not the only Belgian who can play. In Diagram 161 is a shot made by Ludo Dielis. We all try maximum English shots into the corner, end rail first, but how many of us would think of doing it here? After hitting the red, the cueball, because of its spin, went "uphill" to score on the white. A clever concept.

Back to Ceulemans. Against Rini van Bracht of Holland he uncorked the umbrella shot in Diagram 162. It is a fairly well-known pattern (No. 169 in *Byrne's Standard Book*), but the fact that the red ball is not in the corner adds to the difficulty. Van Bracht was so impressed that Ceulemans made it

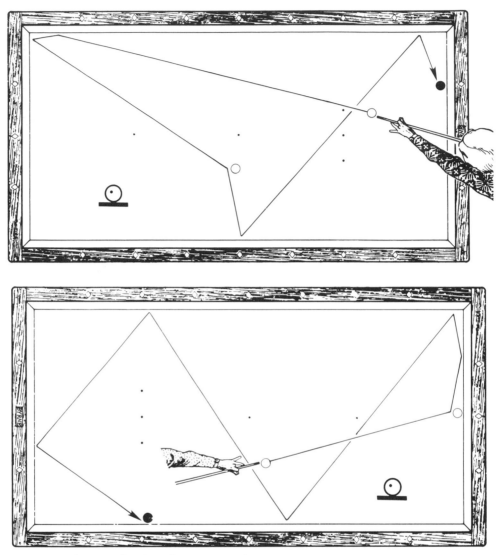

Diagrams 162 and 163: Shots from master play

under pressure that he left his chair and congratulated him with a handshake. The crowd loved the gesture of sportsmanship, though it may have been a hustle.

If you try the idea in Diagram 163, remember that in Germany the cloth was brand new, which resulted in some unexpected angles, especially "backups," as off the fifth rail in this shot.

Next are five shots from the 1986 world tournament in Las Vegas.

The position in Diagram 164, left, faced Ceulemans during his game with Argentina's Doyharzabal. I think every American player would have played this twice-across shot by staying "above" the balls, shooting first to X, then back to Y and over to Z. But the world champion went "below" the balls as shown, using a lot of speed.

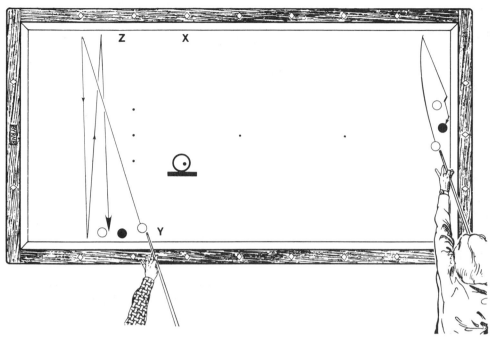

Diagram 164. Shots from master play

Former world champion Nobuaki Kobayashi of Japan came up with the shot in Diagram 164, right, during his game with Torbjörn Blomdahl of Sweden. After pondering his options, he decided to elevate his cue about 30 degrees and shoot the half-massé as shown. He made it perfectly.

One of the surprises of the tournament was 24-year-old Marco Zanetti of Italy, the first player from his country to qualify for the World. For many years he has spent his annual vacations in Vienna, Austria, studying straight billiards, balkline, and one cushion with the great Heinrich Weingartner. Only after reaching world class in those games did he turn his attention to three cushion, and he surprised many observers by how quickly he mastered it. A handsome, personable player who speaks excellent English, he made several lovely massé shots in Las Vegas. One I saw is given in Diagram 165. Soft speed was used, and the cueball landed lightly on the second object ball.

Carlos Hallon of the United States came up with the great shot in Diagram 166 in his win over Mohamed Al Mashak of Egypt. I might have thought of the pattern if the white ball had been on the rail, but it never occurred to me that it is also a good choice when it is five or ten inches off the rail. The action off the second and third rails on the slippery cloth was beautiful.

The most sensational shot I saw in Las Vegas, and the one requiring the most imagination, was pulled off by the 23-year-old Blomdahl against Al Gilbert. How many players would have thought of the amazing time shot in

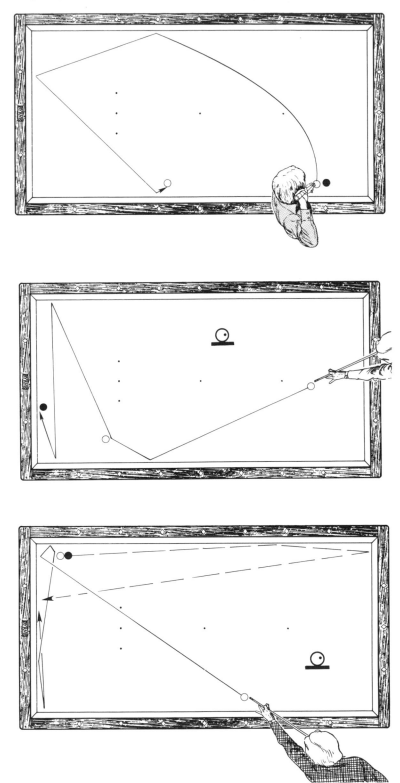

Diagram 167? Hitting enough white ball to make the cueball double the end rail helped kill its speed and keep it at the far end of the table, thus increasing its chances of being in the vicinity of the returning red ball. Some luck was needed with the shot because it was not possible for Blomdahl to predict exactly where the point would be scored. Some spectators remembered the shot a little differently, but I have drawn it as Blomdahl explained it to me after the game.

H. L. Mencken, the so-called Sage of Baltimore, once suggested that a person should change jobs every ten years for the sake of variety and to avoid getting into a rut. The same advice can be offered to billiard players. Three cushion is largely a game of imagination—you have to visualize the shot before you can make it—and if you play with the same people all the time you rarely get a new idea.

I spent most of 1987 in Denver, and played billiards several times a week at the Denver Athletic Club, a labyrinthine red-brick facility that covers half a city block. The DAC has the best billiard room I've ever seen, a paneled beauty containing three snooker tables, two ten-foot pool tables, and five old-style billiard tables kept in perfect condition.

Crossing cues with the DAC regulars has reminded me of shots I had nearly forgotten, taught me some new ones, and shown me that certain shots aren't quite as hard as I thought.

Jerry Karsh, former president of the Billiard Federation of the U.S.A., doesn't shrink from the shot in Diagram 168. Because the cueball is still spinning when it reaches the third rail, the red ball is bigger than it looks.

Leonard Williams is an uncanny instinct player and one of the best freewheelers in the business. When he gets rolling you might as well sit

Diagram 168. Shots from master play

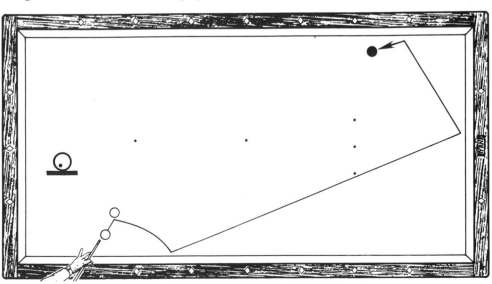

down and order lunch. He is especially good on shots of the up-and-down variety and jumps on them as if they were pigeons. Look at the shot in Diagram 169. I saw Williams make that twice in the same game.

Don Buckmaster loves umbrella shots. A guideline he uses in calculating them involves assuming that the angle the cueball will take off the second rail is 45 degrees. In Diagram 170 the cueball is at the right. To find the point of aim for an umbrella shot, first lay your cue along the edge of the red ball at a 45-degree angle, as shown by the dashed line. Note that the line crosses the third rail 2.7 diamonds from the corner. Now use the standard diamond system as if you were trying to hit 2.7 on the third rail. In the given

Diagrams 169 and 170: Shots from master play

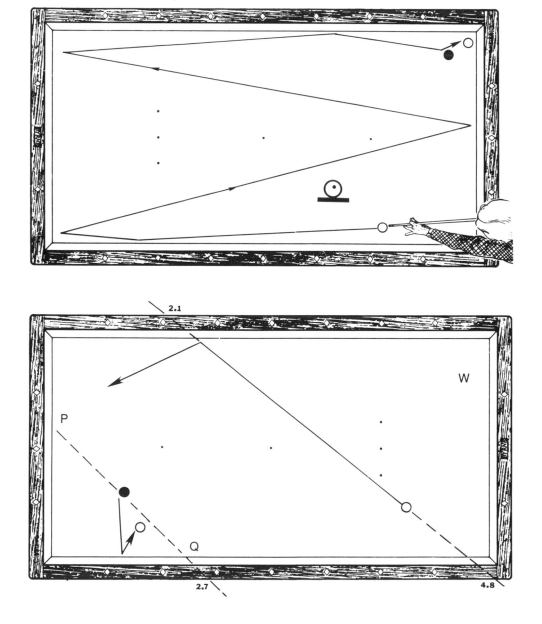

position, shooting out of 4.8 to 2.1 would do it. The 45-degree approximation works well enough for most positions, but sometimes must be modified. If the cueball is at W, for example, an adjustment has to be made.

Peter Undiks is another dangerous DAC player. In the 1984 Denver Open, he was faced with the tough position in Diagram 171. It took real imagination to come up with the shot he made.

In the 1986 Denver Open, I left former national champion Harry Sims of California the position in Diagram 172. If either object ball were frozen, a force follow could be tried. Or if either ball were a little farther off the rail, ticky-ticks would come into consideration. I probably would have tried some sort of up-and-down shot. Harry's elegant solution is shown. We all know the pattern, but how many of us would think of it with the object balls so far from the end rail?

The 1985 Denver Open sported such luminaries as world champion Raymond Ceulemans and French champion Richard Bitalis. Bitalis made the

Diagrams 171 and 172: Shots from master play

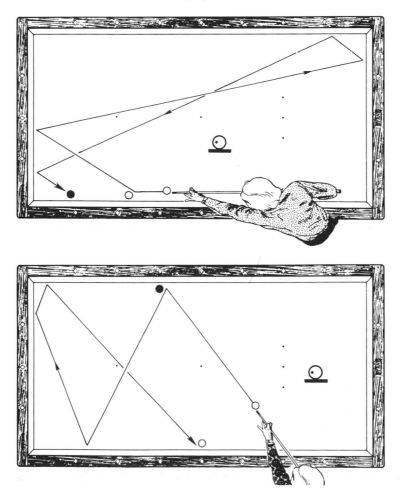

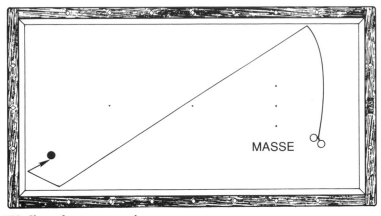

Diagram 173. Shots from master play

remarkable massé in Diagram 173 against Ceulemans. He elevated his cue about 50 degrees and shot just barely hard enough to reach the red, which left the other cueball far away in case of a miss.

It never would have occurred to me to use a massé just to get a good angle on a backup.

The moral of the story is simple. If you can get away from the same old players once in a while, do it.

Now for some shots from the legendary Gus Copulos, who died in 1981 at the age of 87.

Gus was one of the inventors of the diamond system, particularly the so-called "plus two" system, and in the 1920s he was one of the most feared opponents in the country. He had a plus score against Willie Hoppe, and once scored 50 points against him in only 19 innings. He ran a 17 in the National League in 1924, 22 in an exhibition, and a remarkable 16 in call-shot three cushion, where you have to call every rail and kiss.

In March 1977 a three-cushion tournament was held at Brunswick Billiards in Los Angeles that was named after Gus Copulos. When the event was over, Gus stepped to the table at the urging of the people who knew him and began "fooling around." In the span of 20 minutes he dazzled everyone who was lucky enough to have remained in the room. He demonstrated one shot after another that most of us had never seen before. I don't know if he invented them or not, but he sure shot them as if he owned them. He was 83 years old at the time.

The diagrams show the shots I remember him executing on that memorable evening. I hope they will help the younger generation of players remember one of the giants of the Golden Age.

Diagram 174. Who but Gus would play the shot this way? With no English and a high ball, the cueball goes very long. To prove the superiority of the shot over other ways of playing it, he made it several times with the white ball in various positions along the rail.

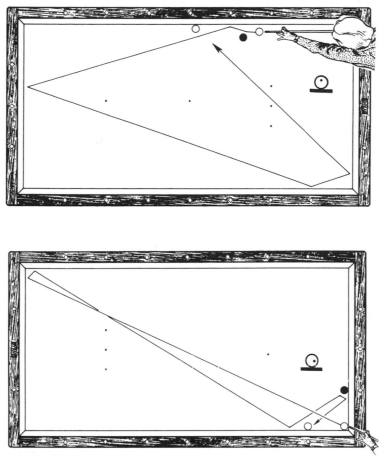

Diagrams 174 and 175: Shots from master play

Diagram 175. A beautiful idea, and not as hard as it looks. After hitting three rails, the cueball misses the white, returning to the white off the red. Related positions come up in games, so it is well to remember the pattern. In a sense it is a two-way shot, because if the cueball feathers the white on the way to the red the point still counts.

Diagram 176. On most tables, a double-the-rail shot wouldn't work in this position. Gus played the shot softly with no English, as diagrammed. The shot can't be made with the cueball much farther to the right because of the English the cueball would pick up coming out of the corner.

Diagram 177. There certainly doesn't seem to be any way of playing a backup ticky in this position, but Gus did it by using high ball and some right English. The cueball, at least when he stroked it, popped off the third rail at a surprisingly steep angle.

Diagram 178. A beautiful kiss-back pattern. The balls are frozen on the three end-rail diamonds. Shoot at the white with low left English, angling the line of aim slightly into the cushion. The idea is to have the white bounce off the side rail and collide with the cueball at the position of the dashed

Diagrams 176, 177, and 178: Shots from master play

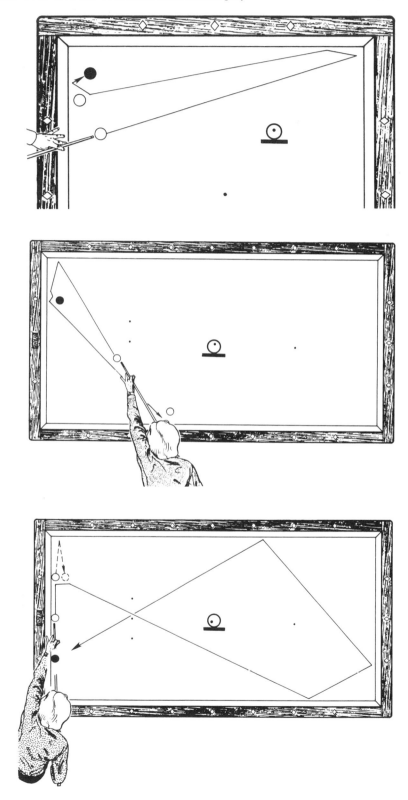

ball, sending the cueball around the table to score on the red. It's easier, of course, with the red big in the corner and the white closer to the other corner, but Gus shot it as shown.

Diagram 179. It was a pleasure to see an octogenarian step up and make a stroke like this. I've drawn it with an open bridge on the player's hand because a downward stroke is needed. Angle the line of aim just enough to miss the kiss and follow straight through.

The final four shots in this section are from Juan Navarra of Argentina, long one of the premiere players in South America. He demonstrated them in 1983 after an exhibition in Novato, Calif.

Consider Diagram 180. The red ball is in a position that can't be reached with a normal shot. With running English you would be lucky to get to point A on the third rail and D on the fourth. In billiard jargon, you can't get long enough. What else is there? If the cueball was a little farther from the end rail you could go thin off the white to point F, then zigzag up the table to

Diagrams 179 and 180: Shots from master play

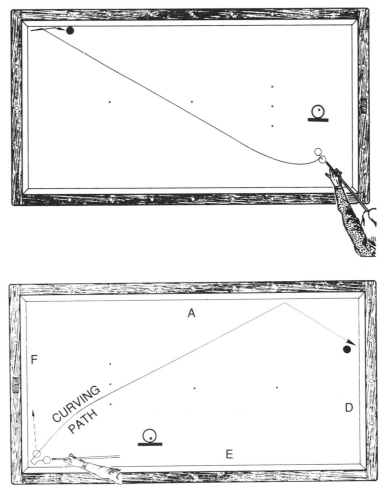

the red. Or you might try a feather-thin hit off the red. Navarra's trick is to hit the white thin as shown with plenty of draw and just a hair of running English. Because the first two rails are hit immediately, the draw doesn't take effect until after the cueball has left the corner, bending the cueball into a "longer" path. The dashed line is there to emphasize how thin you have to hit the object ball. The shot is also good if the second object ball is at E or F. Shoot with crisp speed.

In Diagram 181 the shot would be a cinch if the first object ball was a little farther from the rail. As it is, even an extremely thin hit will bring the cueball in short of the red, and the white is so close to the rail it's hard to get through the hole without a kiss. So play the kiss! Feather the white, and as soon as the cueball comes off the rail it hits the white again and is realigned into a scoring path as shown. Stroked with the proper speed, the white often banks across the table (dashed line) to a favorable position near the corner at A.

The position in Diagram 182 is nasty. Trying to shoot a natural off the white with right-hand English will likely result in a foul or a miscue; besides, even if you manage to get a clean hit, you probably won't hit the right-hand short rail far enough from the corner to score. Navarra makes the shot easily by "bending the ball." Elevate the butt of your cue to about 15 or 20 degrees and use extreme follow and just a touch of right English. Aim so that it looks like you aren't hitting enough of the white. The cueball comes off the first rail at the wrong angle, then bends forward. Don't shoot hard, or the curve won't take place soon enough. The cueball should die near the red.

In Diagram 183 is a cute kiss shot. Every three-cushion player knows the general pattern: rail first with reverse English to the first ball, then spin out of the corner. In the diagram, though, the second ball is in the wrong

Diagram 181. Shots from master play

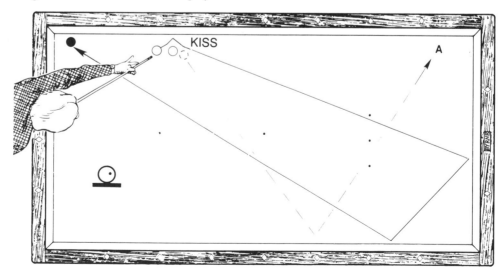

place. With practice, you can learn to drive the red into the white, moving the white into the path of the cueball.

Diagrams 182 and 183: Shots from master play

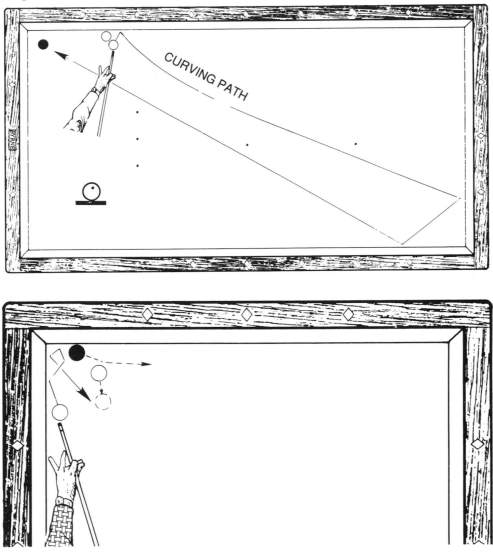

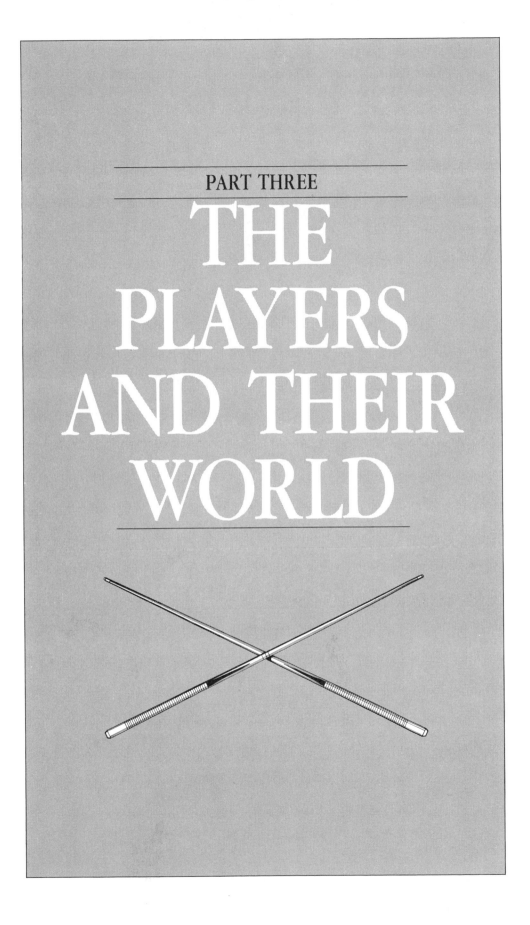

PART THREE

THE PLAYERS AND THEIR WORLD

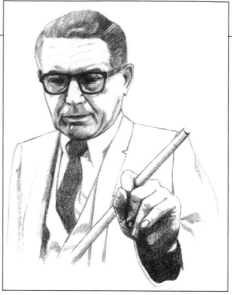

Pencil renderings by Cynthia Nelms

Danny McGoorty
and the Hustler's Life

Excerpted from **MCGOORTY, A Billiard Hustler's Life**,
by Danny McGoorty, as told to Robert Byrne
(Citadel Press, 1984).

McGoorty is speaking:

FOR AS LONG AS I CAN REMEMBER, I HAVE BEEN FASCINATED BY pool and billiards. As a kid in San Francisco I used to skip school a week at a time and do nothing but stare through the windows of pool halls. What I saw was paradise: guys who didn't have to wear knickers and who played pool all the time, laughing and gambling and shooting the bull.

There was a Greek joint on Kearny Street that I liked because I could sometimes sneak in and take a few shots—this was in 1916 when I was 15 years old. Usually before I had time to chalk my cue the chief Greek had me by the seat of the pants and was slinging me through the door. I can still feel myself getting hoisted by the crotch and run across the floor on my tiptoes. In a year's time I gave that Greek a hell of a workout. He finally said I could stay, but only if I was with my father. My father had left the picture years before—he just walked out, my mother said—so I had to spend my school lunch money to hire one, which was no problem. Every pool hall had a regular staff of old geezers sitting around soaking up the heat, and whenever I showed up with change jingling in my pocket a dozen of them got to their feet and volunteered to be Dad.

My mother had a traveling job and couldn't keep track of me, so she sent me to Chicago to live with my two spinster aunts, who were supposed to provide me with a proper home life. I don't know what my mother should have done, but sending me to Chicago was not it. Compared to Chicago, San Francisco was like kindergarten.

For a couple of years I had my aunts believing that I was spending all my time looking for work. They even gave me carfare to make it easier. They smartened up finally and told me I had to get a job and quit making excuses. They were not going to keep on supporting me, they said, if I was idling instead of choosing a career.

Pool hustler, that's the career I was choosing. Playing pool was the only thing I liked to do. Day and night I studied the top Chicago players, watching how they controlled the cue ball, how they played defense, how they hustled babies like me. There was money being made, a lot of money, and I was sure I could get good enough to win my share if I worked at it. I kept my eyes open and practiced every day until my arm felt like lead. I don't call that idling.

I took odd jobs now and then but I always hated working. A job to me is . . . well, it is an invasion of privacy. Getting blasted out of bed by an alarm clock so you can go somewhere and do things you don't want to do, that's not my idea of living. Assembling parts and selling soda pop and delivering packages struck me as ridiculous and always made me feel like a member of the Albanian Bowling Team.

One thing puzzled me. Why do people feel so bad when they lose a job? It made me feel happy as hell, and I always celebrated with a few drinks. When you *get* a job, that's when you should have the long face. You need a few drinks then, too.

My aunts gave up on me and eventually kicked me out, just like my mother had before them. I didn't care. I couldn't stay sober and I couldn't keep a job, but I had improved so much as a player I could make almost as much hustling as I could working. I moved to a cheap rooming house. I remember waking up there one afternoon with a terrific hangover. I stared at the ceiling for a long time, and then I said to myself: "McGoorty, what you have turned out to be is a two-bit, drunken pool hustler." That didn't depress me at all. Listen, I was glad to have a profession.

By 1923 the Chicago hustlers were leaving me alone. I was one of them. I got a run of 72 in rack pool. That may not sound like much today, but it was on a 5-by-10-foot table with 4-inch corner pockets. The world tournament record on that kind of equipment at the time was only 85. The tables they use today are smaller and easier, which changes the game entirely. The promoters did that to get more scoring and longer runs for the spectators.

Pool hustling is a very tough line of work. If you expect to make anything you not only have to be a good player, you have to be a psychologist, an actor and a thief, as well. Marks aren't easy to find, and once you get hold of one it's quite an art to make the biggest possible score. There are a million tricks. You never make a tough shot, unless you can make it look lucky. Miscuing five times in a game of rotation is par . . . not just any miscue, but one that leaves no shot. Miscuing properly, so that it looks accidental and so that the cue ball goes where you want it to, is a good weapon.

Sometimes it's hard to get a mark to play for money at all. A way that worked many times for me was to offer to play a game of rotation "for fun." I would set him up for the 1-ball, and when he made it I would hand him a dime, saying that by "for fun" I meant a dime on every odd ball. Not many guys could turn down that dime. Once they took it, naturally I could go ahead and make the rest of the odd balls.

We would make up all kinds of games to get people started. "You make the 1-ball in the side pocket, and I'll make 50 balls in the other five pockets." That sounds like a terrific handicap, but it really isn't; you just make sure you never leave the guy a decent shot at the one in the side. If he gets his ball close to the hole, you just knock it away. But it sounds great—50 balls to one.

There were a lot of places to hustle pool in Chicago in the 1920's, a dozen big rooms in the Loop alone within walking distance of each other. There were quite a few of us hustling at the same time, so we had to split up and spread out. You couldn't just hang around or the cops would pick you up for vagrancy. You had to keep on the go. I used to carry a newspaper with a few classified ads circled to make it look like I was looking for a job. Standing on a street corner I always had a bus transfer. We kept going from room to room. In case a mark wandered into a place when we weren't there, one of our bird dogs would phone us. I had a bird dog in every action room who would tip me off for small change. If a couple of us were sitting in a room when a mark walked in we would sometimes draw straws to see who got first crack at him.

There is a risk in losing the first game on purpose because the guy might quit and walk out with your money. I soon learned to win the first game as if by luck—then I could throw a game on the *other* guy's money.

In 3-cushion billiards a good way to hide part of your skill is to shoot into kisses. Try to get a kiss off the second or third rail. Not even good players will suspect you are doing it on purpose.

On the road you can work a room for two or three days if you aren't known, or even longer, climbing up to the better players as the bums drop off. When you get to the local shark you still have to hide your stuff because the guys you beat the day before might wise up and get a little unhappy if they see your true speed.

Some hustlers I knew were terrific actors. You would swear they were drunk, or sick or just learning to play. Tugboat Whaley used to put on rain gear, rubber hat and all, and say he was a tugboat captain who just retired on a nice pension that he didn't know how to spend. Marks figured there was no way he could have been practicing pool on a tugboat.

Wimpy Lassiter, before the tournament prizes got big enough to lure him into the limelight, dressed up like a hillbilly, with bib overalls and a piece of straw a foot long hanging off his lip. That was his hustle, pretending he just fell off a hay wagon. The straw hat he wore was a work of art, the way it had been chewed on . . . just enough to fringe it. The hillbilly lingo he used, though, was no con; that was the way he really did talk.

Just as much money changes hands between the "sweaters"—the spectators—as between the players, and that is where the real treachery comes in, because the players might be in cahoots. When the best player throws the game it is called a "dump." The next level is the "double dump," when the mark thinks he is in on a fix and then is double-crossed. There is even the "double double dump," when a guy thinks he has been let in on a plan to double-cross a mark who thinks he knows a fix is on, only to be double-crossed himself. All the players do is make the game come out so that their secret partner on the sidelines wins his bet. I've seen guys go to a lot of trouble to arrange a fix only to find out that *they* were the marks all along.

But using secret partners and pulling dumps and double dumps—lemonading, we called it—is bunco, real con. In fact, all hustling where you hide your speed is stealing. I gave it up as soon as I could afford to, which was about 30 years later. I guess it was true what they said about me—too lazy to work and too yellow to steal.

Early in my career I had the misfortune of taking a few drinks in the middle of a tough game and then coming from behind to win. I thought I had stumbled onto a secret: I could settle my nerves by swilling a little giggle soup. I started going to the can in the middle of every game to suck on a bottle. Before long I was overdoing it, and when I came out of the can I could hardly remember what table I was playing on. My nerves were settled, yeah, but I didn't know what the hell I was doing.

Plenty of times I played for money when I didn't have any, which is called playing on your nerve. When you do that you absolutely have to win. You can't show any mercy or give the other guy any chance at all. All good hustlers and tournament players have the killer instinct, and the way they get it is by playing on their nerve a few times. A lot of good players never get to the top because when they get ahead in a game they start feeling sorry for their opponent. They ease up on him instead of kicking him when he is down. Players who do that have never had to play for their breakfast. You've got to look at it this way: If you are playing your grandmother a 50-point game, try to beat her 50−0. If you are ahead 49−3, try to keep her from getting four. Try to hate her. It helps to hate whoever you are playing. I don't know how much talent I have, but I have a lot of natural hate.

Pool halls were crowded during the Depression. The more people lost their jobs, the more there were to hang around. They didn't have much money, but there were a lot of them. POOL HALL BURNS DOWN—5,000 MEN HOMELESS. That was a common joke, but it wasn't funny. Times got awful tough. Guys were sleeping five and six to a two-bit room. One guy would rent the room and the other guys would sit in the lobby till the desk clerk looked the other way so they could run up the stairs. When I took jobs in pool halls I always hated closing the place at night because it meant waking guys up and throwing them out in the cold.

By 1940 I was almost starving to death. Hustlers used to wait in line in the pool rooms, day after day, hoping a mark would walk in. Sometimes they were reduced to hustling each other. Then World War II started and things changed for the better. I was in California at the time and I noticed the way guys started showing up with money in their pockets. People had jobs again, good paying jobs. By 1942 I was surrounded by marks and saps and suckers of all descriptions. They were pouring into California from all over, looking for people to lose their money to. Kids on the way to Japan figured they were going to get killed, so they didn't care about money at all. I patriotically took it from them so they wouldn't spend it on ladies-of-the-night and get terrible diseases. World War II was like spending four years with your hands in other people's pockets. It was a field day, a thieves' paradise. Then the war ended. The jobs dried up, the servicemen disappeared, and I lost quite a bit on horses and boxers. It was fun while it lasted.

Danny McGoorty died in 1970 at the age of 69.

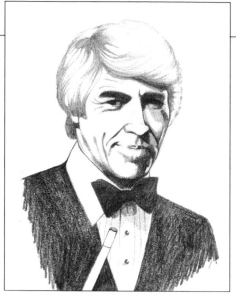

The Filming of
The Baltimore Bullet

IT WAS WEIRD THAT DAY IN 1979 SEEING STEVE MIZERAK, ONE of the most gifted pool players in all of human history, losing twelve games of nine ball in a row. Twelve times he forked over a stack of lovely green money. In the background, digging into their billfolds and shaking their heads in disgust, were five of the hottest sticks in the game, "Machine Gun" Lou Butera, Richie Florence, Alan Hopkins, Pete Margo, and Jim Mataya. Mataya didn't seem as unhappy as the others—attached to the elbow of his green tuxedo was a smashing blonde in a clinging sheath.

The weirdness lay not so much in the multiple drubbings absorbed by Mizerak as in the flaws in his opponent's technique. Overall, he was everybody's idea of a pool shark, a lanky man with cool gray eyes, a sinister smile, a lined face, and a way of circling the table like a wolf smelling a kill. But his stance was odd. There was something less than silky-smooth about his stroke. He lacked the uncanny accuracy and cueball control of the master he was fleecing.

"You're playing great tonight, Nick," Mizerak said, screwing his cue apart to show he had had enough. "You should have been in the last tournament. You would have taken my trophy away from me, too."

The man called Nick, his eyes slits, deftly flicked through the currency. His voice dripped derision: "If I wanted a tin cup I'd buy one. Cash is where it's at."

Director Robert (*The Heart Is a Lonely Hunter*) Ellis Miller jumped to his feet, pleased with the twelfth and final take of a scene in a movie called *The Baltimore Bullet*, a FilmFair Production. "Cut! Excellent! Print it!"

This was the land of make-believe, specifically MGM's Sound Stage 25 in Southern California. Inside the blimp-hangar of a building wizards had conjured up a cocktail lounge and pool tournament arena, with walls decorated by framed photos of billiard champions, jockeys, and boxers. The set is a glorified replica of the roadhouse in Johnston City, Ill., where a decade earlier a series of pool tournaments was held.

The movie stars James (*The Muppet Movie*) Coburn as Nick Casey, world's most feared money player, Bruce (*How the West Was Won*) Boxleitner as his partner on the road, and Ronee Blakely (she was Barbara Jean in *Nashville*), who hocks her pet horse so that Nick can challenge a high-roller in a white suit played by Omar Sharif (you loved him in *The Mysterious Island of Captain Nemo*). That's Coburn in the drawing on the facing page.

When the scene was described "in the can," the set was invaded by an army of supervisors, assistants, technicians, advisers, electricians, carpenters, gaffers, and grips. Cinematographer James (*The China Syndrome*) Crabe bent over the pool table with a light meter. A makeup man dabbed at Coburn's cheek with a power puff. Special effects men pushed through the crowd with smudge pots. "Hey," somebody complained, "do we really need so much smoke? This isn't a war movie." Lights, microphone booms, and camera dollies were repositioned. Instructions were issued in movieland code. A wardrobe assistant tugged at Jim Mataya's collar, straightening his killer-butterfly bow tie, while a prop man traded his glass of beer for one with a fresher looking head. Through gritted teeth the normally unflappable Mataya whispered: "I don't know what the hell is going on."

What was going on was the production of a movie that the producers hoped would match *The Hustler* as a popular favorite and moneymaker. But *The Baltimore Bullet* is upbeat, a comic romp through the pocket-billiard subculture, far different in flavor than the 1961 Paul Newman classic, which dwelt on sleaze, suicide, and the breaking of thumbs. Released in 1980, it sank without a trace in the United States, though it did fairly well overseas.

That pool hustling can be fun and that some hustlers treat life as a kind of continuous party were discoveries made by the film's producer, a former professional dancer named John Brascia, while touring the country with a pool-hustling friend. There is the changing scenery, he found, the memorable characters, the celebrating that follows a big win, the gambling, girl-chasing, horseplay, con games, and storytelling. There is the thrill of victory and the thrill of defeat—agony comes only when there is no game at all.

Brascia decided that it was time for a new movie about the game and its practitioners that would make people laugh and feel good and that would, in addition, display the amazing skill possessed by the masters of the green cloth. So he sat down at a typewriter and wrote his first screenplay. Five years, rejections, and rewrites later he got lucky. FilmFair, one of the world's largest makers of television commercials, had decided to expand into feature films. After considering some 70 novels and scripts, the firm picked Brascia's "action comedy," about two pool hustlers who can't seem to stay out of trouble and who are sustained on the road by dreams of the big score that may be just around the corner.

In a fine piece of Hollywood chutzpah, ten of the top pool players in the country were cast as themselves, namely, Lou Butera, Irving Crane, Richie Florence, Alan Hopkins, Pete Margo, Ray Martin, Jim Mataya, Steve Mizerak, Jim Rempe, and Mike Sigel. The names are listed in alphabetical order to avoid the further breaking of thumbs. Each man believes he is the best and has a closetful of backers and trophies to prove it.

FilmFair, having set up a $4.5 million budget, brought in the best technical talent available in an effort to assure a box-office hit.

Supporting actors, bit players, and even extras were chosen with special care. Particularly effective as a fearsome but bungling thug was Jack O'Halloran, a six-foot-six, 250-pound monster-man fondly remembered for the way he threw Gene Wilder off a train in *The Silver Streak*. O'Halloran was a respected heavyweight boxer. His 1972 bashing-match with Ken Norton, which he narrowly lost by decision, was so thoroughly enjoyed that the crowd showered the ring with $600 in change. Another show-stealer was Michael Lerner, who was Jack Ruby in *Ruby and Oswald* and Pierre Salinger in *The Missiles of October*. He attacked the role of pool tournament promoter Paulie Jansco with wonderful gusto and bluster.

The flavor of the film is at its most pungent in a banquet scene that takes place at the start of what is called the All-Around World Championship Pool Hustlers' Tournament. The raucous crowd suggests a Mad Hatter's Tea Party, a Damon Runyon convention, a reunion of high-rollers, sharks, pimps, touts, and con artists accompanied by their mouthpieces, molls, and mistresses. Extras, when asked how to dress for the scene, were told to strive for "a polyester look." The tournament promoter (Lerner) has to shout to make his announcements heard over the tumult: "This year, for the first time, the tournament will be covered by television. (*Cheers from the crowd*) Which means I don't want no obscene crap. (*Boos*) Furthermore, all players have got to wear tuxedos." "Who's getting married?" someone calls from the floor. "We came here to play pool!" (*Cheers*) Lerner ignores the remark and goes on at the top of his voice: "Anybody who doesn't have a tuxedo can rent one from me for fifteen bucks a day. And don't bother asking for credit. I'm not a finance company."

Here the camera closes in on Coburn, who says to Carolina Red (Blakely), "Paulie had open heart surgery last year. They couldn't find it."

Nick "The Baltimore Bullet" Casey (Coburn) is a professional hustler who sneers at tournaments and their nickel-and-dime prizes. He is at the banquet because the mysterious "Deacon" (Omar Sharif) will play him a match for $40,000 only if he wins a tournament.

"Well, well, well," says real-life champion Steve Mizerak when he spots Coburn, "if it isn't Nick Casey. What are you doing here? I thought you didn't play for tin cups." He lifts a glass of beer and adds, "Or are you just showing off?" The gesture and words will be familiar to anyone who has seen the television commerical Mizerak did for the Miller Brewing Company, the one in which he shoots three successive trick shots and lifts a glass of beer off the table just in time for a speeding cueball to pass underneath.

New York's Pete Margo has a line at the banquet, too. Elfin and button-bright, he introduces his stakehorse, a man named Robin Hood because "he steals from the rich . . . and keeps it," to Carolina Red, calling her "de only skoit I know who shoots as good as a man."

The banquet is followed by the tournament. As luck and writer-producer Brascia would have it, the championship game is between Coburn and Boxleitner, best friends and partners in a thousand scams on the road, who have always avoided playing each other. At last the gamblers in the stands and the world at large will find out which one is best.

Or will they? Before the game begins O'Halloran slams Coburn against the men's room wall and tells him to throw the game because his money is on the kid, and before it ends there is a raid by the massed forces of the state police and the F.B.I., just as a hoodlum after the prize fund blows the office safe with a grossly excessive charge of explosives, while a short distance away Sharif and his henchmen . . . But leave us not give it all away.

Any misgivings the director might have had about integrating ten pool sharks into his cast were dispelled early by the naturalness of the players. "They were easy to work with," Robert Ellis Miller said. "I told them to be themselves, and they were. They are vivid people with a fresh, raw quality. They are performers themselves, you know, used to the limelight, not bothered by cameras and audiences. It was wonderful to look through the lens and see ten of the best pool players in the country having such a good time."

When James Coburn is making a movie, he's usually glad when the 12-hour shooting sessions are over so he can hop into his Ferrari 308 GTS and speed home to his snooker table and his collection of exotic drums, gongs, and flutes. *The Baltimore Bullet* started out the same way. In his words: "After twenty-seven days of filming it was becoming awfully hard work. Then the players arrived and turned everything into a party. It was fun all day long! They are fascinating characters, full of personality, confidence, and style, not sallow, poolhall stereotypes. I could hardly wait to get to work in the morning."

Getting to work in the morning was a bizarre concept to the players, most of whom hadn't held a conventional job in years. Breakfasttime is considered the middle of the night. "Don't worry," Pete Margo said on his first day, yawning at noon, "we'll all be here at 7:00 on the dot every day. Vanity will drive us from our beds. We are dying to be in a movie."

The set was a bar, so the players felt at home. A stagehand warned Richie Florence not to put his foot too heavily on the brass rail because it was only lightly tacked in place, and somebody else asked him if it wasn't a little early in the day to be drinking. "Of course not," he replied, lifting his glass in a mock toast, "it's cocktail time in Bangkok."

"But look at your eyes!" laughed Margo. "You look like you've been playing Dracula and overfed."

Most of the scenes involving the players call for them to be holding glasses as well as cues, and the property master was kept busy pouring beer.

Rudy Oliver, a black local player whose white tuxedo looked as though it would glow in the dark, raised his glass in the air after every take and announced: "I drank my prop."

It was a party, all right, and the long breaks between scenes were filled with card games, pool games, jokes, and storytelling. Irving Crane, a dignified man who has been playing world-class pool for 45 years and who claims, along with Mizerak and Willie Mosconi, never to have been a hustler, was an endless supplier of anecdotes. Like Bobby Fischer, he remembers every game he ever played: "I once ran 150 and out in a straight pool tournament against Joe 'The Butcher' Balsis. Two years later we met again and he ran 150 and out on me. When the last ball dropped he turned and said, 'Let that be a lesson to you.'"

Ray Martin described winning the 1971 World Tournament in Los Angeles, which is best remembered for the earthquake that struck during the preliminary rounds. Dallas West, according to Martin, packed up and went home to Rockford, Ill., despite being undefeated, remarking, "Who needs this?" In the same tournament Steve Cook lost a game because a tremor readjusted the balls, leaving him without a shot.

Mike Sigel fondly recalled a hustler he used to travel with who would "do anything to suck a guy into a game. To make himself look stupid, he'd walk into a poolroom wearing a baseball cap backwards. To look handicapped, he'd have a fake cast put on his arm. He once won $1,300 from a guy who had never lost more than $150 in his life by making himself look like an awkward clown at the beginning. He did that by walking into a joint carrying a sack of groceries, bumping into a pool table, and spilling oranges all over the floor."

Alan Hopkins is built like a college halfback. When he wasn't killing time playing nine ball or flipping coins for $100 bets he was playing backgammon with Jim Mataya for $25 a point. High stakes don't bother him. "I won $90,000 a couple of months ago playing pool with a guy back East. You know what he did when it was over? Took me out and bought me dinner. Now that's class. He had no chance to win because I am the best in the business. Who is better? If you know, give him my address and tell him to bring money. I like money. I have a wife, kid, house, and three cars to support."

But Mataya feels that *he* is the best in the business. "Nobody will play me. I have a standing offer to play anybody any pool game for any amount. Most of the players here should come to me for coaching."

Lou Butera admitted that he was not in top form at the moment, but claimed that when he is he "murders everybody. I kill them, and it doesn't take me all day to do it, either. I once ran 150 balls in 21 minutes. When I'm right, anybody who plays me needs one of these . . ." As he spoke he tore sheets from a pad of Death Certificates.

Jim Rempe, who once won 41 straight matches of tournament nine ball, will gaze quietly into anyone's eyes and state that he is the greatest player in the world. So will Mike Sigel. Both claim to have won more tournaments in the last four years than anyone else. Rempe elaborated: "A lot of players will *say* they are the best, but only a few of us *know* we are the best."

Michael Lerner, laughing after hearing so many conflicting claims of supremacy, said "Amazing! These guys have bigger egos than us actors!"

"Steve Mizerak is a great player," Irving Crane said with his customary calm, "no doubt about it. So is Ray Martin. The cockiness of the young players shouldn't surprise anybody. You've got to believe you're the best if you want to be the best. All of the players here are excellent, with hardly an eyelash of difference between them, especially when they are playing on a 4½-by-9-foot table with loose pockets. On an old 5-by-10-foot table with tight pockets, though, I would win. I don't *think* I would win, I *know* I would win."

Rempe shrugged off Crane's remarks. "I've heard all that stuff about how tough the old-time 5 × 10s were and about how Ralph Greenleaf and Willie Mosconi were the greatest players of all time. Not true. The greatest players of all time are the ones playing now. And among the greatest, I am the greatest."

Living legend Willie Mosconi, resplendent in a gray suit with matching gray hair, was on the set to play the role of a television commentator. He was asked whether he thought he was a greater player than the late legend Ralph Greenleaf. He refused to answer. "But I will say this. When he lost a game people said it was because he was drunk. What they forget is that when he won a game he was drunk, too."

When the day came for the players to leave the set it was like the break-up of a summer camp. The normally wary hustlers were shaking hands and embracing the actors, crew, and staff as if they had been friends for years. They were actually being *affectionate.* James Coburn embarrassed Jim Rempe by kissing him on both cheeks. Bruce Boxleitner put his arms around the shoulders of two players, jostled them, and said, "I love you guys."

The production was heading for New Orleans with Omar Sharif, where the schedule called for shooting the windows and doors out of a car with a shotgun, dropping a casket out of a hearse, knocking a cop off his horse, wrecking a string of parked cars, and shearing off a fire hydrant. The players wanted to go along.

"*Please* take us," Pete Margo begged the producer and the director. "Find something more for us to do. We'll pay! We'll pay good money!" His offer declined with thanks, he threw up his hands and turned away. His voice was full of sadness when he said: "You are about to see ten pool players cry."

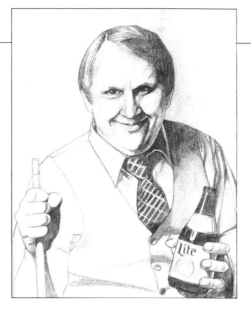

A Visit with
Steve Mizerak

LATE ONE AFTERNOON IN 1979, STEVE "SCHOOLTEACHER" MIZ-erak was relaxing in a chair beside a hotel swimming pool in Culver City, Calif. Mizerak is a burly man with thin sandy hair, not as slender and speedy as he was 20 years earlier when he was pursuing basketballs through various New Jersey gymnasiums. He leaned forward and spoke carefully, making sure his words were being taken down without error.

"When you shoot a lot of pool in bars," he said, "you want to stay fast and loose. You don't want to get filled up. That's why I drink Lite beer from Miller. It has a third less calories than their regular beer, and it's less filling. Plus the taste is great. And even though a lot of people don't think pool is strenuous, let me tell you something. You can work up a real good thirst even when you're just showing off."

He was responding, of course, to a request for a recitation of his lines from his famous commercial, the first ever to appear on network television featuring a pool champion. He had no trouble remembering the words—after all, the commercial required the amazing total of 191 takes to give it the desired look of casual perfection. "I knocked the glass of beer over twice," Mizerak recalls with a smile, "ruining the cloth. Thank God the cueball never hit the bottle, which had a hand-painted label and was worth $250."

The commercial made Mizerak one of the few pool players who enjoys some degree of public recognition. He is getting more requests for appearances and exhibitions than ever before. "Things were beginning to open up even before the ad came along. Several big tournaments and television events are in the works. I think the next couple of years are going to be crucial. If the right decisions are made, a lot of top players are finally going to make some decent money."

It's about time. Mizerak and dozens of championship-caliber pool players have devoted a large portion of their lives acquiring a skill that has been very poorly rewarded, especially when contrasted with the cash and glory that are routinely heaped upon stars of the so-called major sports. In Mizerak's case, the skill began to be acquired when he was only four years old in his father's pool room in Perth Amboy, N.J. Steve Senior, still a fine player of both pool and billiards, showed him the fundamentals, and after a couple of years it was evident that the lad had a remarkable aptitude for the game. He got his first run of 50 in straight pool when he was 11 years old, his first run of 100 two years later.

He wasn't a "pool freak" exactly, because he was interested in many sports and games, particularly basketball. A typical day for him in grade school and high school was to rush home after basketball practice to put in a couple of hours at the pool table. He won the city championship at 13, and in the following six years did well in the tough New Jersey State Championship, never finishing lower than third despite having to contend with such players as Jack Breit and Danny Gartner. His first national-class tournament was a 75-point, single elimination straight pool affair called the Television Tournament of Champions. Irving Crane finished first, Steve Mizerak second. Once he hit the winner's circle, tournament victories began piling up steadily. Only 43 years old in 1990, his list of first-, second-, and third-place finishes is already as impressive as anyone who has ever picked up a cue. Whenever he enters a tournament, no matter what the competition or the style of play, he is always a good bet to win, place, or show. Straight pool and nine ball are his best games, but he also plays top-class snooker and billiards. A few years ago he traveled to England and beat John Spencer three games of snooker, though he modestly dismisses the feat as a fluke. He feels that the British snooker masters in a long match on

6-by-12-foot tables with tight pockets will defeat the best American pool specialists. As for billiards: "I'm about ready to enter one of the three-cushion tournaments. If I practice for a couple of months I think I could give Jimmie Cattrano all he could handle."

Practicing, though, is not something he enjoys doing. "I've never been the type of guy who could set up certain shots and shoot them over and over. I'd rather give a room player a tremendous handicap than practice by myself."

Early in his career, particularly during his teens, he worked on his game three or four hours a day. Now he doesn't need that much time to stay sharp. When an important tournament is coming up he practices two or three hours a day for two or three weeks. He stops playing entirely four or five days before it starts, then practices again the day before.

His cue is a 21-ounce Balabushka with a 12¾ mm tip. It is 58¾ inches long (Steve himself is 6 feet 1 inch tall), almost two inches longer than average. He feels that the extra length is very helpful on shots that require a long reach.

Mizerak has come a long way since the time he got his first run of 100 on his home table. A few years ago at the Golden Cue in Queens he ran 179 and out in one game and began the next game with a run of 90. His personal high run of 285 continuously came in a match against Ray Martin. He'd rank among the world's richest men if trophies were money.

In action, he stalks the table with intense concentration, pocketing balls with such a methodical rhythm that many of his fans refer to him as Mizerak the Machine.

One of the remarkable things about his early success as a player is that he was always either a full-time student or teacher. Unlike most of the other top players, he has never been a road hustler. After graduating from Alabama's Athens College, where he majored in education, history, and psychology, in June 1967, he went to work in September as a seventh-grade teacher at William C. McGinnis junior high school in his hometown, a job he held until 1981, when he decided to pursue his pool career full time. In 1989 he gave more than 60 exhibitions, many for corporate clients like Miller, IBM, K-Mart, and Philip Morris.

The pool scene has changed considerably over Mizerak's professional career. "In the old days there was more unity among the players and promoters. Things were tough and we all tried to help each other. Now everybody is trying to cut everybody else's throat. If we could stop that I think we could all make some money. If pool doesn't break through into the big time in the next two or three years, I don't think it ever will. We've got to capitalize on the opportunities we have now and try to eliminate the jealousy and bickering. With all the big deals that are brewing, the money may soon be at hand."

Pool tournaments are a form of show business, whether they are televised or not, and show business is based on the star system. Who are the stars that will replace Willie Mosconi and Minnesota Fats as drawing cards for the general public? So far only one name has clearly emerged: Mizerak the Machine.

Making a
How-to-play-pool
Videotape

A TIP OF MY HAT TO STEVE MIZERAK, FOR I KNOW NOW HOW hard it must have been to film that Miller Lite commercial in which he made three trick shots in a row with no camera cutaways, all the while delivering a timed, memorized spiel in a voice that sounded fresh and enthusiastic. I know now why it took 191 takes to get it right.

I also have new respect for the smiling mannequins who read the evening news on television. They may be bubbleheads in real life, but they can do something that is harder than it looks: talk for minutes on end without stumbling over their tongues . . . and make it look effortless.

The way I gained these profound insights is by spending three days in 1986 on a Hollywood sound stage making two one-hour videotapes on how to play pool. For three days I was pampered as if I were Shirley Temple, handed a drink of ice water or a peeled grape whenever I put out my hand, and given a fresh shirt whenever the sweat stains got too gross. There was even a full-time makeup lady (never had she faced such a challenge) following me around with a powder puff to keep the shine off my nose and the dew off my lip.

Not that I wasn't slapped around a bit. "Cut!" the director would yell, jumping from his chair and pulling great gobs of hair from his head. "Bob, for God's sake, try to keep in mind that you are giving away priceless jewels, not conducting an autopsy or doing your ironing!" At other times he would say things like, "Excellent, Bob! Now let's try it again without the lisp." Or: "Look into the camera! The camera is your friend. It is a nice camera. Don't keep glancing off to one side as if you expect the cops to break in." At one point the producer, after a seemingly endless series of takes of a simple follow shot, came out of the control room and said gravely, "It would help if you could make a shot straight into the pocket." I found that highly amusing and felt for a moment like banking him into the side.

If everybody would simply have gone away and left me alone, I could have made all the demonstration shots with soporific regularity. If they had given me a typewriter in a soundproof room, I could have written a narrative for someone else to read that would have shimmered with elegance and grace. If I could have sat under a shade tree and answered questions about the game, I could have impressed a Shakespearean with my eloquence and diction. But to shoot pool, explain what I'm doing and look cheerful under 100-degree lights with cameras over my head, off my elbow, and in my face, well, that's another rack of balls entirely.

The idea of making a videotape on the game had been festering in my mind for years, in fact, since *Byrne's Standard Book* came out in 1978. Some things are well explained by a diagram in a book, but others can be understood only by seeing them demonstrated—by seeing the dynamics involved. A tape to go with the book, I felt, would be the ideal combination for a player wanting to improve.

I talked to people in the video business every year or so, and while they were interested in the idea of a first-class pool tape, one that would make full use of such things as overhead cameras, slow motion, and electronic enhancements, they weren't interested *enough*. I didn't want to make an imitation of the pool tapes already on the market, which have a kind of home-movie quality about them, with ad-lib narrative, a camera fixed on a tripod, and inadequate lighting. What I had in mind would cost a bit of money, and I simply never was able to make the right connection . . . until I found Cimarron Productions in Hollywood.

Cimarron is best known for making trailers (previews), television ad spots for feature films (Star Trek V, The Fly II, Rain Man), and movies on the making of movies. The company was looking into producing something of its own for the growing video market. Head man Chris Arnold likes the game and was more than a little interested in the potential for a well-produced and well-organized tape on how to play pool.

I was asked to submit an outline of what I thought the tape should cover, then a full script including suggestions for camera angles and graphics. The script took me a week to write and ran 50 typewritten pages.

One of the factors that prompted Cimarron (and its Premiere Home Video division) to proceed was the successful completion by Disney Studios of the film *The Color of Money*, which by all indications would bring thousands of new people to the game; it was a good business gamble to have an instructional tape ready for them.

When I arrived in Hollywood, I found out just how small I think. I thought we could go to a pool hall with a couple of cameramen and a floodlight and get enough footage in a day for two one-hour tapes. I thought I could simply use a sketch pad and a felt tip pen when something technical had to be explained. Given the teaching I have done, I thought the narration would be a piece of cake. I was wrong. It was staggering to see the amount of time and money Cimarron had already invested in the project and what was planned for the coming week.

The flaw in my approach was that I was thinking of the hardcore pool market, the one that can be reached through the pool publications and the retail stores that specialize in the paraphernalia of the game. Unfortunately, that isn't a big enough market to justify the cost of making a fully professional tape. Of the some 30 million people in the country who play pool at least occasionally, less than 5 per cent (I'm just guessing here) are aware of such things as billiard magazines, billiard retail stores, or nine-ball tournaments. A much bigger market had to be targeted, and that meant sporting goods stores and videotape rental outlets, neither of which currently stock pool tapes. To crack the huge videotape rental market would require a product made to the highest technical standards. While sales of a thousand or two is all that can be expected for inexpensively made tapes aimed at the hardcore fans, Cimarron would have to move at least 20,000 to break even.

Instead of a pad and pencil, I was presented with a 2-by-4-foot, steel-backed demonstration board covered with pool cloth and designed to look exactly like a real table. A set of miniature pool balls, sliced in half and backed with magnet-backed plastic pieces (i.e. arrows, circles, lines, and so on), had been made up for use as visual aids when explaining such things as the geometry of massé shots. My pointer would be a tiny cue. All together, it was the niftiest teaching aid I'd ever seen.

I was shown nearly finished four-color art, flashy and dynamic, that would be used for brochures, for advertising, and for the videocassette's slipcover. I was shown blueprints for the set, which was being built on a Burbank soundstage. I met a bewildering number of people who seemed to know me and who already had been working on the project. I began to feel like the guy in the one-act play *The Actor's Nightmare*, who keeps finding himself in the middle of plays where everybody knows what's going on but him.

Saturday and Sunday were devoted to rehearsing on a practice table in the showroom of Billiard Library in Long Beach. The sessions enabled director Arnold to prepare a detailed "shooting script," with directions for each camera. When the narration mentioned my grip hand or the cueball or an object ball at the far end of the table, the cameramen had to be prepared to swing to the right place. If I left one scene to the right, I had to enter the next one from the left so that the action flowed smoothly. If a shot on the table was reshown from another camera, it had to be planned so that it didn't seem to "flip over," like the reverse angle replays in football.

Then there was the need to tear the script apart and paste it together out of sequence so that time could be saved by minimizing the number of camera and lighting setups. Everything at the demonstration board, for example, would be taped at once. It was an enormous amount of work for Arnold, who worked nights as well as days.

The set was built in a cavernous soundstage by a crew of stagehands and carpenters. The walls, which appear on camera to be divided by brick columns, were decorated by historical billiard art from the collection of Terry Moldenhauer. (On the second day I leaned against one of the "brick" columns and almost brought the whole set down.) Moldenhauer's Triple A Billiards in North Hollywood set up the table, a massive Trafalgar model made by World of Leisure. I asked that it be covered with Simonis because a fast, slippery cloth provides a better showcase for curving cueballs.

When I arrived for work at seven-thirty Tuesday morning, I found a scene I wouldn't forget. There were at least a dozen people on the set: gaffers, grips, cameramen, assistants of one kind or another, and several whose functions I couldn't begin to guess. In the control room were people with titles like audio mixer, video engineer, tape engineer, and script girl.

Three cameras were ready, two mounted on wheeled dollies and a third on a 20-foot boom that could be put at any point in space and at the same time aim the lens in any direction. The mass of wires trailing behind the cameras and lights formed an incredible tangle of spaghetti on the floor. A stack of "idiot cards" had been prepared for me to glance at when my mind went blank, which was often. After my face had been lathered with cosmetics, making me look like a cross between Abraham Lincoln and Tuesday Weld, we were ready to roll.

Shooting the first scene was a harbinger of things to come. All I had to do was enter through a door, look around admiringly at the set, screw my cue together, break the balls, turn to a certain camera, and introduce myself. It must have taken an hour to get everything right—my movements and words, the camera angles, the lights. All through the day the shooting was bedeviled by the gremlins that apparently are routine in the movie business: a plane roars overhead, a light inexplicably goes out, somebody coughs or kicks a plug from a wall socket, the performer mispronounces his own name, a camera runs out of tape or film. Even the simplest scene has to be repeated over and over to make sure there is one satisfactory "take."

It was twelve hours a day under broiling lights, three days in a row. The heat affected the behavior of the performer as well as the balls. I had unexpected trouble with some of the easiest shots in the game, like the hustler's trick of keeping a ball on the rail by moistening the contact point between two frozen balls; when I raised my fingertip to my mouth, my tongue felt as dry as a blotter, and when I did manage to transfer some saliva to the ball, the lights dried it off before I could bend over and shoot. Another problem was demonstrating the throw effect because the brand new balls were so clean, hot, and dry there was little friction between them, and the throw was hard for the cameras to pick up. I eventually decided to cheat by chalking the contact points. Then the balls threw off line . . . and how!

All problems were solved one way or another. I tried to make everybody feel at home by acting temperamental and difficult, at one point demanding a larger dressing room and a mobile home in which I could sulk. The requests were refused. On the third day I arrived wearing sunglasses and an ascot. The crew rewarded me by pasting a star on my plastic cup.

When videotaping was finished, the postproduction phase began. Specialists went to work adding music, editing the raw footage into a finished product, picking the best takes from the three cameras, adding slow motion and special effects (when I indicate a line on the table with my cue, it appears on the screen through the miracle of modern electronics), and integrating footage from other sources.

I was changed by the experience. For one thing, I will never again make fun of Gerald Ford, who was criticized for being unable to chew gum and walk down the street at the same time. Sounds easy, but try it when the cameras are rolling.

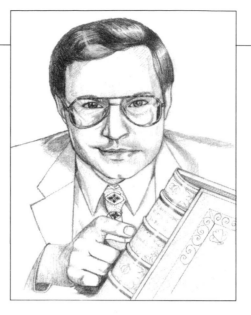

Michael Shamos,
Billiard Archivist

ASK THE NEXT 500 PEOPLE YOU MEET IN A POOL HALL, A BIL-
liard supply store, or a billard industry convention if they've ever
heard of Mike Shamos. You'll be lucky to find half a dozen who have.
Yet Michael Ian Shamos of Pittsburgh, Pa., is one of the most important
people in the game. What he is doing, what he has already done, will
last as long as there *is* a game.

In 1983 he bought the largest collection of billiard books, graphics,
and memorabilia in the world from Dick Meyers of San Pedro, Calif.
Since then he has not only tremendously expanded it, spending some
$125,000 in the effort, but has spent hundreds and hundreds of hours
creating a computer-based index, a cataloger's dream, that makes the
entire colossal mass accessible.

The Meyers collection was called Billiard Archives and was assembled during a decade of buying, selling, and trading. Shamos kept the
name but dropped the "s" because, as he rightly points out, there is
only one. When I visited him a couple of years ago I was astounded at

what he had achieved. I'm a bit of a collector myself of billiardiana, but the scope, breadth, and depth of the Billiard Archive and the way it is organized staggered me. The major holdings include 600 books, 600 pieces of art, 1,000 photographs, 250 postcards, thousands of newspaper clippings, and hundreds of artifacts. By comparison, the Library of Congress has about 250 books on billiards.

Shamos was born in 1947, wears glasses, and is ten pounds heavier than he'd like to be. What struck me most when I first met him and his wife, Julie, were his enthusiasm, his energy, and his intelligence. He's friendly, he's good company, and he's a veritable fountain of curious lore on any number of subjects. He's the only guy I know who can be called a polymath, which my American Heritage Dictionary defines as "a person of great or varied learning."

The man himself is as amazing as his Archive. He majored in physics at Princeton and went to graduate school at Yale, Duquesne, American University, and Vassar, getting a Ph.D. in computer science, a law degree, and five other degrees. He taught computer science for six years at Carnegie-Mellon University and formed two highly successful software companies, Unilogic and Lexeme, both of which were sold in 1987. He speaks several languages, including Russian. He is an expert on such unlikely and unrelated subjects as fur, election fraud, and bagpipes. (He recently put together a meticulously researched dictionary of 6,500 bagpipe tunes.) Name any subject and he'll talk about it.

When he took me through his home in Pittsburgh, showing me his collection—which covers the walls and fills several rooms—he did it with the pleasure of a boy in a toy store . . . and with the pride of a man who not only *owns* the toy store but who invented the *concept* of toy stores. There was an almost tangible excitement in the air as well—at last he was able to show the results of his labors to someone touched by the same obscure obsession, while for my part I was seeing something I thought existed only in heaven. Everything was beautifully displayed, framed, cased, and shelved, and what wasn't on view was stored in a seemingly endless array of map drawers, bookcases, and filing cabinets. I stayed overnight in a spare room; it was like sleeping at a shrine.

The only collection I have seen that is halfway comparable is the one assembled by Heinrich Weingartner in Vienna, Austria, which emphasizes European material.

I sat with Shamos in a darkened upstairs room in front of a computer monitor while he demonstrated the indexing system. With the help of a modem, he was able to access a high-speed computer in his office building downtown. I asked various questions. When was plastic first used for balls? When was Willie Hoppe born? When did rubber cushions come in? The answers were on the screen in seconds. And not only the answers: the system also showed what filing cabinet and what drawer and what folder contained additional information.

I asked him what he had on Jake Schaefer, Jr., the great balkline champion. Soon a screenful of references to clippings and magazines appeared, then another screenful, then another, each reference briefly summarizing what could be found in various folders. I finally told him to stop the scrolling and simply ask the computer *how many* references to Schaefer there were. The answer was 610.

I asked for references to myself and was stunned to see more than 50! Everything I had written about the game, or had been written about me, over a 25-year span was there, itemized and labeled. Yes, I thought, there is a Billiard God, I am staring into its face, and it has me by the lapels.

Other sports and games would be lucky to have a man as tireless and productive. Single-handedly, he has captured and catalogued the long history of the game and is making it available to devotees and historians. He can demonstrate with documents and graphics just how broad and rich and colorful the game's history is. Particularly impressive is his ability to show how much attention artists through the centuries have devoted to billiard themes—from the early engravers to Van Gogh and Currier and Ives. One of his recent tasks has been to reduce the Archive's major holdings to color slides so that researchers don't have to paw over fragile originals. A by-product of the effort is a series of 300 slides that can be used for a lecture on the evolution of the game and the roles it has played in society.

Other recent projects include a massive glossary of pool, billiard, and snooker terms, complete with anecdotes and quotes from writers ancient and modern, which should be ready for publication in 1991. In 1987 Shamos toured Asia carrying a card on which was written in Chinese: "This man is interested in books on billiards. Please sell him some. Thank you." The result was the acquisition of 21 books in Japanese, 23 in Chinese, 1 in Thai, and 10 in English, increasing the Archive's book collection by 10 percent.

I sent a list of questions to Shamos about the Archive and about the origin of his interest in the game. The answers came back in narrative form.

"I was introduced to billiard games by my father, who was a three-cushion player in college and is still very good. I played incessantly as a student at Princeton, to the detriment of my studies, and was taught three cushion by a grizzled old security guard there. Taking the academic approach to billiards as I did with most subjects, I started to research what had been written about the game and found a small shelf of books in the university library, including Daly's Billiard Book. I was astounded to learn that it was actually possible to control all three balls in billiards. With Daly's help, I began to learn.

"I tried every old bookstore I could find to buy a copy of Daly, but failed. This started my lifelong quest for antique billiard books, which becomes more of a disease each year.

"I drove to Elizabeth, N.J., to buy a Palmer cue, and I eventually won the university three-cushion championship two years running and took first place at the Association of College Unions Northeast Regional tournament in 1968. Despite those victories, I'm really not very good. At best, I average about .500 in three cushion. In straight pool, my high run is a solidly mediocre 42.

"I spent a dangerously large amount of time at McGirr's in New York learning the game from hustlers, including Jack Collar and the infamous Bandito Cortes. My big moment at McGirr's came when a hustler I had never seen before challenged me to a game of three cushion for money. I told him I had to warm up first. I spotted the balls, happened to run seven, and said to him: 'I'm ready. Twenty points for fifty bucks.' He said, 'Maybe some other time.'

"In 1975 I began to search actively for old billiard books by visiting antiquarian bookstores and requesting mail-order searches. One correspondent offered me an old engraving showing two French soldiers playing billiards and I learned that there was a whole unexplored world of collecting to be investigated, namely billiard art. I wrote for a catalog of Billiard Archives in California, but didn't buy anything because I felt the prices were too high.

"By 1983, when I had managed to scrounge together about 75 books and a handful of prints, I saw that the entire Billiard Archives was for sale. I wrote for the inventory and was amazed at what it contained—almost all of the books I had been wanting for years—almost 1,000 lot numbers and more than 3,000 individual items, including many oddities like cigar box labels, medals, postage stamps, billiard cloth sample books, and sheet music of billiard songs.

"I begged my wife to let me make an offer. I was sure I wouldn't be the successful bidder, but I found out later that I was the only one to make a serious bid. What I acquired was the antique material, the name, and the goodwill of Billiard Archives. Modern material, such as posters and books in print, were sold separately by Dick Meyers to Bob Baskin, who started a mail-order company called the Billiard Library.

"My idea was to create a research collection. I felt strongly that someone knowledgeable about billiards must do it or a gap would be left in our understanding of the history of the game. If the collection were to go to a large institution, like a public library or the Smithsonian, it would likely be stored away in boxes and not be studied, maintained, or expanded. I took up the challenge and formed a Pennsylvania non-profit organization called the Billiard Archive (singular), registering its purpose with the Secretary of the Commonwealth as 'The collection, retention, and historical research of billiard memorabilia and the promotion of the study of the game of billiards and its variations.' The Billiard Archive collects; it is not in the business of selling its holdings.

"I have vastly expanded the Meyers collection, particularly in the area of old prints, books published before 1850, and foreign material. The current value of the collection, measured at what I paid for it, is about $125,000. It is housed in my home and protected by a state-of-the-art security system. All of my free time goes into searching for new items and cataloging what I already have.

"Anyone of serious purpose may see the collection by appointment. Because of the irreplaceable nature of the holdings, their value and importance to billiard history, visits are carefully controlled. As curator, I will help locate records and use the index. Nothing may be borrowed, but photocopies of uncopyrighted material will be made for small fees, which go toward expanding the collection. We have assisted movie companies, authors, architects, and even a department store that wanted a window with a billiard theme. American Gramaphone Records recently issued a volume of Mozart with a reproduction of a print from the Archive showing billiards being played in Vienna around 1790.

"I solicit donations of funds or, preferably, billiard memorabilia. Unfortunately, while the Archive is nonprofit, gifts are not tax-deductible according to current interpretations of the I.R.S. Future expansion does not entirely depend on the charity of billiard enthusiasts. Fine or important items are bought, if necessary.

"I can't overemphasize the importance of the print collection. Reliable written accounts of billiard playing do not appear before the 1770s. We have engravings, however, that show the game a hundred years earlier. Printed accounts dwell on billiards as played by the rich and powerful; artwork shows us a cross section of social classes.

"The Archive has a number of items I consider gems, including:

- An exquisitely bound edition of White's 1807 book with a fore-edge painting by an English caricaturist. When the book is closed the pages look gilded. When it is opened or the pages rolled, a painted billiard scene miraculously appears;
- An 1875 handwritten French manuscript with watercolor plates and fine binding;
- The 1694 engraving by Trouvain showing Louis XIV at the table;
- The original 1827 French edition of Mingaud's book on trick shots with hand-colored illustrations;
- An engraving by Van Lochom dated 1640 showing gnomes playing billiards on a table with detachable rails.

"Because library material is useless without an index (an item that can't be found might as well not exist), and because of my background in computer science, I resolved that the Billiard Archive would have the best index and cataloging system of any collection in the world. Every item received is indexed according to type, author or artist, title, size, year, source, and descriptive key words. By rapid computer searching we can find, for example, the name of the room in which Cannefax became so angry about his match with Hoppe that he slashed the cloth with a knife (Mussey's in Chicago, 1925), or when eight-inch balklines (soon abandoned) were introduced. Such searches take less than a minute. I will answer any historical question that is accompanied by a contribution of $10, refundable if the answer is not found. (The Billiard Archive, 605 Devonshire St., Pittsburgh, Pa. 15213.)

"The index can also be used to produce fully typeset bibliographies and catalogs of any part of the collection.

"As extensive as the Archive is, many items are still needed. I am anxious to acquire fine prints of all eras, but especially before 1860. Of the eight Currier and Ives engravings related to billiards, I have only five. The Archive needs more foreign material, postcards, movie stills, photographs of players and halls, and rule books published between 1915 and 1945.

"It's fun to dream about what the Billiard Archive could do if resources were unlimited:

- Set up a public museum of billiards. The idea has been under discussion for decades, but nobody is willing to commit the necessary funds;
- Publish a complete color catalog of the collection;
- Make low-cost reproductions available;
- Maintain a staff to search for and catalog material;

- Sponsor research into the history of billiard games and publish the results;
- Assist in keeping the game popular."

That's Mike Shamos. Billiards is one of the oldest and most popular games in the world and deserves more than it has received from historians, libraries, museums, and even its own manufacturers and suppliers.

Working behind the scenes and with a low profile, Mike Shamos has managed to salvage much of the game's heritage all by himself. Think of what he could do with industry support.

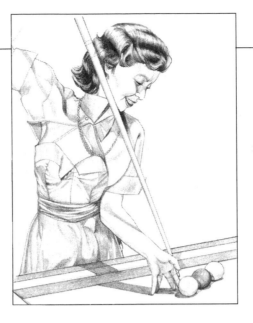

Masako Katsura,
Japan's Shooting Star

S HE WAS A MERE SLIP OF A THING, 5 FEET TALL AND 96 POUNDS, but what a phenomenal billiard player! She was petite, polite, precise, feminine, charming, modest, entrancing, and a scoring machine unlike any other. Masako Katsura of Tokyo burst on the American scene in 1951 at the age of 37 and proved that size, strength, and sex need have nothing to do with cue skill.

She had proved the point in Japan, pounding on the male players as if they were so many temple gongs, and male-dominant Japan had a hard time accepting it. American men as well still have trouble accepting defeat at the hands of a woman.

When she showed up at the 924 Club at Fifth and Market in San Francisco—a wonderfully ornate and atmospheric billiard parlor that Willie Hoppe had called the best room in the country when it opened in 1909—Katsura caused a sensation. Owner Welker Cochran, many times world champion in balkline and three cushion, was stunned. He had heard about her from servicemen returning from Japan, but discounted the rumors of her skill until he could watch her play in person. When he did, he came out of retirement and played a series of three-cushion matches with her in Portland, Kansas City, Chicago, Detroit, New York, and San Francisco. A year later he staged a world tournament to see how she'd do against Hoppe, Irving Crane, Joe Chamaco, and other world-class professionals.

"She constantly amazes me," Cochran told a reporter in Kansas City, "by the shots she makes and by her little inventions which compensate for her lack of size. I knew five minutes after seeing her play in my home, even though she hadn't touched a cue in six months, that she was one of the really great. She has the touch that makes what she does appear so simple and yet is so extremely difficult." He pointed out that she not only had a flawless stroke, but perfect rhythm and surprising power. "Billiards," Miss Katsura said to the reporter in broken English, "is fun."

Cochran began a week's matches with her in San Francisco by trying to give her 10 points in 40. She dropped that, however, when it became quite obvious that she needed no help. At the halfway mark, Katsura trailed only 320–331. "She's playing phenomenal billiards," Cochran said. "I don't mean phenomenal for a woman, but for anybody."

The old pro eventually took the series, scoring 543 to Katsura's 480 in only 491 innings. That a woman, a diminutive one at that and one who had never before concentrated on three cushion, could average .978 against one of the greatest players in history, had aficionados humming.

Sportswriter Jimmy Cannon described the New York match, which took place in a green-curtained alcove at the long-gone Elkan's at Broadway and 44th. Cochran won the first game 50–34 in 45 innings, Katsura the second 50–39 in 39 innings.

"The audience," Cannon wrote, "small but intense, was awed by Miss Katsura's talents. The woman hurried around in a rapid walk. Once she had surveyed the table, crinkling her forehead in meditation, there was no hesitation. The stroke was quick but unhurried. People gazed at her through the faint nicotine haze with reverence. When Miss Katsura missed a shot, her eyes pulled into a squint, her face frozen into a grimace of regret. When she scored, the people applauded. Then her smile exposed her gold-guarded teeth."

"If you eliminate three cushion," Cochran claimed, "I don't think you could find five people in the world who could beat her. Her best games are straight rail and balkline, but she'll be the three-cushion champion of the world in time. She has one of the best strokes I've ever seen, and she shoots as well left-handed as right-handed."

I can vouch for her ambidexterity. When I arrived in San Francisco in 1954, I watched her practice straight-rail billiards by first running 75 points right-handed, then 75 left-handed. Danny McGoorty phrased it with his characteristic color: "She flips the cue back and forth like a chopstick."

After managing to split ten exhibition games with her, McGoorty said, "I played hard and threw her all the dirtiest stuff I knew. If you had the slightest idea of easing up because she was only a cute little girl, you were dead. She would murder you. She would take those balls away from you and stick them right up your pooper. She was tough to play because of the way the crowd reacted to her. Every time she shot, the whole crowd leaned, hoping she would score the point. When I shot, they leaned the other way. Her short angles were terrific. On short angles she had everybody out looking for work."

She used to practice for four hours every morning at the 924 Club and sometimes still was there when I arrived for my lunch break. She was mesmerizing, with her quick step, her dartlike stroke, her fluent style. I felt I could at least avoid disgrace against her in three cushion, and once worked up the nerve to ask her for a game. She agreed, and even though I played as well as I was capable of, she swept past me as if I were treading water. Losing a game to her remains a highlight of my life.

She was a legend in Japan long before she married American serviceman Vernon Greenleaf (no relation to Ralph) and moved to the United States. She was born in 1914 and took up billiards at age 14 when her oldest sister married a room owner. It wasn't long before she was women's champion of Japan in straight rail. After age 19 she confined herself to the men's tournaments and twice was runner-up in the national straight-rail tournament.

International star Kinrey Matsuyama taught her the diamond system in three cushion and watched with pleasure at her rapid progress in that form of the game. In one exhibition before coming to America she had a run of 19.

It was in straight rail that she reached the loftiest heights, many times running 500 and out from the break. In the four-ball version of the game that is popular in Japan, she once ran 10,000 points, an incredible feat that took four and a half hours and involved going around the table 27 times executing the rail nurse.

Two younger sisters, Noriko and Tadako, also won the national women's championship in straight rail. That brother-in-law must have been a heck of a teacher! He coached her and when she was ready he brought men to his billiard parlor to play her. Masako told Cannon: "I practice before parlor open every day for two hours. Every day I practice. Soon I play with many men. Men want to beat me. I play men, six, seven hours a day. Men no like, they do not beat me. If I hit no good, my brother-in-law, after billiard parlor closed, say this shot no good. This shot bad. I make good. He tells me. Not so many good woman player in Japan. I have sister. Very good. Same stroke."

Miss Katsura's debut as a contender for the world three-cushion crown took place in San Francisco in December 1951 in a tournament that was to be Hoppe's last. Katsura's first match was against Crane, who was not just a straight-pool player. Curley Grieve, sports editor of the *San Francisco Examiner*, described the scene: "It was the first time my eyes beheld a woman competing on equal grounds with a man in a world championship sports event. The lady is Miss Masako Katsura of Japan, so small and doll-like she looks like a figurine in her flowing, gold-satin gown.

"She was positively sensational in her opening match. She lost to Irving Crane, but what of it? Her shots were amazing and her behavior unruffled even in the face of disconcerting breaks that included a referee's decision at a crucial, tide-turning point.

"If the gallery had been packed with women, they would have risen to their feet and given her a roaring ovation at the end. She had achieved something historic for her sex. One cannot refrain from lavishing praise on this mite of a creature who asks no mercy of a case-hardened group fighting for their dignity.

"Old billiard followers were in the front-row seats. National picture magazines had a corps of cameramen and writers present. Rugged characters from the pool rooms, unbelieving at first, sat as if awed by the intrusion of such beskirted talent. A half-hundred spectators who couldn't buy seats huddled at the doorway of the draped arena."

Crane built up a lead of 12 points, then began to show the strain as Katsura cut it to 4. Grieve heard a voice behind him say: "Look at Crane, fighting for his life." Then Cochran whispered, "I never thought I'd see this day. She is magnificent." Crane pulled it out, 50–42.

Hoppe won the tournament, losing only to Ray Kilgore and Joe Procita. Katsura finished seventh in the field of ten, beating Kilgore, who was to become world champion the next year, Arthur Rubin, Procita, and Herb Hardt. She lost to her former teacher Matsuyama, who finished second to Hoppe, by a score of 50–48.

Her performance was covered by much of the nation's media. She appeared on the early television show *What's My Line?* In its March 17, 1952, issue, *Time* gave her a full page, saying that "her youth was well-spent." In answer to the question "What is it like to play such a difficult game in front of hundreds of people?" Katsura replied, "I am alone at the table."

Next came the 1953 world tournament in Chicago. Nobody realized it at the time, but it was to be the last United States world tournament of the old professional era. Kilgore edged Jay Bozeman for the title, with Harold Worst, John Fitzpatrick, and the great Zeke Navarra finishing third, fourth, and fifth. Right behind that group were Katsura and Matsuyama. Katsura had impressive wins over Bozeman, Navarra, Joe Chamaco, and Herb Lundberg to finish with a record of 5–5 and a grand average of .830.

She continued to improve, coming in fourth in Buenos Aires the next year in a tournament won by Worst with the Navarra brothers next. That was the end of big-time billiards for more than a decade and it was the end of Masako's career as well.

Talk about lousy timing! Had Katsura reached her peak in the 1920s she would have become rich and famous, as would be the case if she were peaking now. As it was, the game fell dead, and a few years later so did her husband, Hoppe, Cochran, Kilgore, Charlie Peterson, and many of the other old-time champions.

Masako retired from the game and lived in obscurity for many years in Pasadena, Calif., where her neighbors and associates knew nothing of her remarkable history. She occasionally came to San Francisco to visit her niece, and on one of those visits, in 1978, she dropped into the Palace Billiards with her friend Ed Courtney, who later became president of the Billiard Federation of the U.S.A. A three-cushion tournament was under way, a good crowd was on hand, and I asked her if she would step to the table and give a brief demonstration.

"I haven't touched a cue in ten years," she apologized. "What could I do?"

I suggested the rail nurse in straight rail. She agreed to try. Somebody handed her a Schrager cue and I had the extreme pleasure of introducing her to the audience and telling them how lucky they were.

I remember well what she did that night. She put the balls close to the rail and on her third shot was so out of position she had to resort to a short massé. The landing wasn't quite right, and she had to gather the balls again by driving the red four rails, which she did with exquisite perfection. There were no more inaccuracies, and the feel quickly returned to those delicate hands and fingers. When she reached 100 points without a miss she smiled and bowed to the applauding crowd, stepped away from the spotlight, and disappeared forever from the American billiard stage.

Recently her niece arranged for her return to Japan, where she plans to spend the rest of her years with her sister Noriko, who is two years younger than Masako. Noriko also had a fabulous career as a player, accomplishing something that even her more famous sister never quite managed—Noriko won the 1956 *men's* championship of Japan in straight billiards, beating Koya Ogata for the title with a run of 1,850 points in the final game. Noriko took the 1972 *men's* title in four-ball billiards as well, a game in which her high run was 7,825, which took over three hours.

Masako is suffering from a condition that affects her recent memory, but she has lost little of her billiard skills. Noriko reports that she is playing again, and brilliantly, and once she starts practicing she almost has to be pulled away from the table no matter how many hours have gone by.

I wish I could be there to see it . . . and I pray daily to the billiard gods that someone is capturing her on film.

Once I asked her if she were taller than Matsuyama. With a twinkle in her eyes she said, "Yes, but only because I can wear high heels." With or without high heels, she towers over the billiard landscape.

Thank you, Masako, for the pleasure you gave to everyone who crossed your path. Here's to your health.

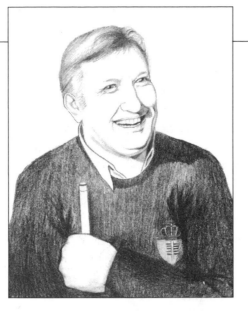

Raymond Ceulemans,
King of World Billiards

NEVER HAS A MAN DOMINATED HIS SPORT THE WAY RAYMOND Ceulemans did between 1962 and 1987. Put the greatest three-cushion billiards players in the world against him and he'd crush them like a handful of potato chips, make them all look like they were in kindergarten, make monkeys of them.

One veteran billiard watcher who has seen the old-time greats perform says that the stocky Belgian is not just the greatest three-cushion player in history, he is the greatest in every phase of the game—the best shotmaker, the best banker, the best defensive player, the best position player; he has the most secure massé stroke, the richest imagination, the widest knowledge, the most delicate control of speed, the deepest concentration, the strongest will to win, and the steadiest nerves.

Pool champion Lou Butera, who saw him play for the first time at the world tournament in Las Vegas in May 1978, said he had never seen such phenomenal precision in his life. "The man is a legend," he said, shaking his head, "and he deserves to be."

A hockey fan from Detroit who was in Las Vegas told me he had switched idols. "Gordie Howe was always my God, but Ceulemans is 40 percent better at what he does than Howe is at what he does."

The tournament win in Las Vegas gave him his 100th major title in the various forms of billiards (he does not play pool or snooker). He has won 43 Belgian, 32 European, and 25 world championships. Not all came in three-cushion events. The man is also one of history's greatest players in balkline, one cushion, and straight billiards. Several times he has won the world pentathlon crown, a competition in which the contestants, at the tables eight to ten hours a day, play grueling round-robins in straight billiards, 18.2 balkline, 28.2 balkline, cushion caroms, and three cushion.

Several European players can give him all he can handle in the so-called "small" billiard games, but in three cushion he became very nearly invincible. "In three cushion," he says, holding out his fist, "I *have* something. The game is in my hand. I know when to defend and when to attack. I know my opponent will eventually make a mistake. As for myself, I feel I can make every shot. There is no particular type of shot that gives me trouble."

No one who saw the dazzling show he put on in Las Vegas can doubt his words. His grand average of 1.678 points per inning set a new standard of excellence that seemed out of reach of everybody but himself. In fact, it is hard to think of any three-cushion record that he doesn't own. One of the oldest marks in the book, the high run of 25 made by Willie Hoppe in an exhibition game in 1918, fell to Ceulemans in 1977. Playing in his room in Mechelen, Belgium, against one of his students, he clicked off an amazing 29 points in a row. Not content with that outburst, he followed it the next two innings with a 2 and an 18—a total of 49 points in 3 innings!

Perhaps the most remarkable thing about Raymond Ceulemans is that 25 years of worldwide acclaim, 25 years of hearing himself described with every imaginable superlative, have not ruined his personality. Here is a man who is practically a national hero in Belgium (once when he was spotted in a theater with his wife the lights were turned up and he was given a standing ovation), yet he is not a braggart, not a poser, not a prima donna. He does not ask for special treatment and he will play anyone for the fun of it. He has the same jovial, good-natured disposition he had at the beginning of his career.

I first met him in 1966 when I helped manage the invitational world tournament in San Francisco in which he made his United States debut. He had won four straight official world tournaments and was up against one of the most powerful fields ever assembled. He impressed everyone with his quick smile and hearty laugh, his cooperativeness and sportsmanship. He got a kick out of the way people mispronounced his name (correct is KOOL-a-munz), and he laughed till tears came to his eyes at some of the stories told to him by the late Danny McGoorty.

Halfway through the tournament, when he was in first place but not shooting quite up to par, the job fell to me to ask him if he had any objection to our replacing the three Italian tables, which were giving several of the players fits with their sharp angles, with three old Brunswicks. I thought I might have a fight on my hands, but he disarmed me by saying that whatever the committee wanted to do was perfectly all right with him.

As it turned out, he finished second in that tournament to 60-year-old Argentinian Enrique Navarra (uncle of the better-known Juan and Zeke Navarra), despite running 16 in the playoff game to decide first place. He was impressively gracious in defeat. He wants to win, but I have the feeling that on the rare occasions when he loses a game he is happy for his opponent because he knows what a thrill it is to beat the world champion.

Once during a European vacation I spent a night in the Belgian town of Grobbendonk, where Ceulemans owned a four-table billiard room-café. When I walked in he was at work as the bartender and sandwich-maker, having a good time joking with his customers. Even though he had made a long car trip earlier in the day he was quick to offer hospitality to a visitor from overseas. He drove me to a restaurant, picked me up when I had finished eating, and when business in his room slacked off late in the evening he screwed his cue together and asked if I wanted to play a game.

He had sensed, correctly, that I lacked the audacity to ask *him* to play. As luck would have it, I got a run of eight at the start and took an early lead, which set the handful of spectators buzzing in Flemish. Ceulemans laughed and said, "I know this guy! He can play!" Well, yes, I can play, but not at his cosmic level. I hardly play well enough to qualify for Belgian citizenship. The point of the story is not that Ceulemans won another international billiard match, but that during the brief time I was ahead he was genuinely excited for me.

Raymond Ceulemans, 52 years old in 1990, is open, accessible, confident, not in the least moody, complicated, or "difficult." He's a man who loves good food, fine beer, and laughter. And he *loves* to play billiards.

After the 1978 Las Vegas tournament and exhibitions in Chicago and Oak Park, Mich., Ceulemans came to San Francisco for a vacation with his wife, Angela, and his two boys, Koen, 17, and Kurt, 15. (Ingrid, 13, and Ann, 11, were in school in Belgium). Bob Bills, owner of Palace Billiards, got the idea of inviting the boys to play in the weekly rapid-fire handicap tournament. I called Ceulemans at his hotel and offered to pick up the boys and deliver them after the tournament so that he and his wife could spend a night on the town together. He liked the idea of the tournament, but wouldn't consider for a minute not being on hand as a spectator. He and his wife not only showed up, they stayed till the bitter end. He rooted for his boys and congratulated every player who made a good shot. He thoroughly enjoyed himself, especially when 15-year-old Kurt took first place, and he got a kick out of the jokes about how the $27 first prize made the lad a professional for life.

It was close to midnight when the tournament ended, but since there were three balls resting quietly on a nearby table he couldn't resist borrowing a cue and running 100 points in straight rail. Someone asked his opinion of another cue—he took it, examined it, then used it to run another 100 points in straight rail. It was then that I noticed his wife was looking very much as though she would like to get some sleep, and I said something sympathetic to her. "It's the same way in Belgium." She laughed with a wave of her hand. "He just *loves* to play."

If you saw Ceulemans walking down the street you would never guess that he was the greatest billiard artist the world has ever seen. He looks more like a football player or a nightclub bouncer, a man in the same general mold as Rocky Marciano. He says he is 40 pounds overweight, perhaps a result of the fare at his billiard cafés in Grobbendonk and Mechelen, where a hundred different kinds of beer are on the shelves.

Even when he steps to a billiard table and addresses the ball there is nothing about his style that suggests brilliance. He is solid and secure rather than flamboyant. When he forms a bridge with his small hands he keeps the fingers together rather than elegantly spread. His stroke is straight and true . . . compact and economical rather than flashy. He plays fast for fun, but in a tournament game he is deliberate and methodical. He plots the course of the balls carefully, but almost always without walking around the table. When he bends over to shoot his body is like a tree trunk or a block of granite; nothing moves except the right arm.

When the balls start rolling, there is no doubt that a master is at work—the speed control, the management of all three balls, the precision hits, the uncanny accuracy and action . . . it all goes together in a magical blend. His manner is so calm and matter-of-fact that you sometimes don't realize how well he is playing unless you keep track of how much faster the points are adding up than the innings.

We can be thankful for those friends who persuaded him to give up soccer as a youth and concentrate on billiards, for which he showed a great affinity from the beginning. His teacher, former Belgian champion Frans Rombouts, turned him loose when he was only 18. "There is nothing more I can teach you, Raymond," said Rombouts. "I can hardly win a game from you anymore. You are on your own."

The precocious student won his first Belgian tournament shortly afterward. I asked him if it was in three cushion. "Of course not. First I had to learn how to play billiards." By that he meant that mastery of straight billiards and balkline are essential for anyone who wants to be tops in three cushion. He makes the point repeatedly. America will never be a threat in international competition, he feels, until its best players add the "small" games to their repertoires. It is the only way to learn subtle nuances in speed and English, to refine your judgment on carom angles, and to accustom yourself to positioning the first object ball.

The young Ceulemans when he turned to three cushion had his countryman Rene Vingerhoedt to contend with, one of the best players in the world at the time. Ceulemans was unable to beat Vingerhoedt in his first two tries for the right to represent Belgium in the European qualifier for the World, but he put up such a struggle that Vingerhoedt saw the handwriting on the wall. Vingerhoedt won the world crown in 1960 and retired to devote himself to exhibitions and teaching. "Otherwise," he said, "I would not have been able to retire as champion. It was obvious to me that Raymond would soon be the best in the world, so I got out while still on top."

In his first appearance in the world tournament in 1962, Ceulemans finished seventh, losing several games by one point. He won his first world crown in three cushion in 1963, averaging an unprecedented 1.302 points per inning. With only one exception in the next 20 years, he was the official world champion, getting stronger and stronger as the years went by.

The lone exception was in 1974, and occurred, strangely, in front of his hometown fans in Antwerp. Nobuake Kobayashi, playing by far the best billiards of his career, nipped the champion by a single point in the last game of the tournament by running six and out.

There was a touching moment at the banquet following the last game. Kobayashi, asked to step to the microphone and say a few words through an interpreter, chose instead to sing a 500-year-old Japanese folk song about the joy that came to a group of villagers when they threw off the oppression of a local governor. He is no threat to Frank Sinatra, but he sang with the sincerity that came with years of finishing second.

The victory by Kobayashi was a bit unsettling to the Belgians. Was the long reign of Ceulemans over at last? Had the hard-working Japanese players finally come into the ascendency?

We know the answers. Ceulemans reasserted himself and won the world title the next five years in a row. He put it well himself when asked to explain that stunning upset in Antwerp:

"I don't know how that happened," he said during an interview on Belgian television. "But the next year the tournament was held in La Paz, Bolivia. There at the closing banquet Kobayashi did not sing."

I once took Ceulemans to a Chinese restaurant in San Francisco. In his fortune cookie was a slip of paper reading: "You are confident of your abilities." He signed it and I put it in a scrapbook.

Proof that he has reason to be confident of his abilities appeared in the way he met the challenge of Torbjörn Blomdahl (see page 215). The young Swedish phenomenon burst onto the scene in impressive style, supplanting the Belgian as world champion in 1988 and 1989. In November and December of 1990, however, Ceulemans won two of the six World Cup tournaments and finished high in the others to once again be crowned king of world billiards. He is not going to hang up his cue peacefully.

And don't forget his two sons. In January of 1991, Kurt Ceulemans, 28 years old, defeated his father three sets to two to take the championship of Belgium!

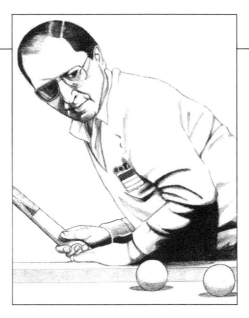

Avelino Rico's
Unforgettable Upset

ASTOUNDING, SHOCKING, THRILLING, UNFORGETTABLE—
the 41st annual three-cushion tournament, sanctioned by the
World Union of Billiards (UMB) and staged by the Billiard Federation
of the United States, was all that and more. When the cheering died
down at the Tropicana Hotel in Las Vegas, May 18, 1986, one of the
most unlikely competitors—Avelino Rico of Madrid, Spain, at 55 the
oldest in the field—was champion of the world. Even in a gambling
town, the odds on Rico at the start were too long to post.

Rico's incredible run of 15-and-out against Belgium's awesome
Raymond Ceulemans in the semifinals when he was trailing 48–35,
followed by his 50–46 win over Swedish prodigy Torbjorn Blomdahl
despite being buried 37–13, made this tournament one of the most
memorable of all time. Not since 1941 has anyone run 15-and-out in a
world tournament (Jake Schaefer did it to Welker Cochran). Never
before has a darkhorse like Rico taken first place. Not since Willie Hoppe
has a man 55 won a world tournament. Never before has anyone

matched Ceulemans's grand average of 1.746 points per inning, and never before has a man as young as Blomdahl, who is only 22, been runner-up.

They'll be talking about this one forever.

When Rico made the last point against Blomdahl, the stocky, bespectacled draftsman—who is relatively unexpressive during a game—thrust his cue into the air in triumph, then threw his arms around his young opponent. As the crowd of 400 stood cheering and applauding, the president of the Spanish Billiard Federation bolted from the stands and wrapped Rico in a bear hug. They were quickly joined by a half-dozen more Spaniards. Looking a bit like a football huddle, they danced and turned and laughed for several minutes in a display of joy that touched everybody in the house.

Even Ceulemans, bitterly disappointed the day before by being denied the crown that would have been his in a round-robin format, embraced Rico and congratulated him.

You almost had to be there to believe it, and even if you were it wasn't easy.

The tournament featured 14 of the world's best players, with a couple of conspicuous omissions. Because of a dispute between the European Confederation and the World Union of Billiards regarding a proposed professional league, Ludo Dielis of Belgium and Richard Bitalis of France didn't participate in the European championship and therefore had no chance to advance to the World. The top four finishers in Europe were Blomdahl, Rico, Marco Zanetti of Italy, and Jorge Thieriaga of Portugal. Ceulemans was eligible as defending world champion. The top three finishers in the United States National were in—Carlos Hallon, Al Gilbert, and Frank Torres. From South America came Galo Legarda of Equador and Luis Doyharzabal of Argentina. Japan's entries were national champion Yoshio Yoshihara and former world champion Nobuaki Kobayashi. Completing the field were two Egyptians, Hisham Saad and Mohamed Al Mashak.

The format of the tournament, the seeding of the players, and the schedule of games were dictated by the UMB. The field was divided into two groups of seven for round-robin play, and the top two finishers in each group went into a single-elimination playoff to determine the ultimate winner. The games were played on three beautiful tables made by Soren Sogard of Denmark in an arena of 400 bleacher seats set up by the Tropicana. Soren Sogard also provided three electronic scoreboards.

The Tropicana recently spent over $80 million on renovations and additions, and the hotel's convention center was a fine place for the tournament. The swimming pool between the two hotel towers is set in a one-acre tropical park, and the gambling casino is so huge and bizarre that in the words of Heinrich Weingartner, balkline champion of Austria, "it goes beyond garish to become beautiful again." There are so many great-looking cocktail waitresses, show girls, and vacationers wandering around that you almost, but not quite, get used to it.

Next to the arena was a room for dealers, where a fourth Soren Sogard table was set up for practicing and exhibitions. Raymond Steylarts of Belgium, world skill-shot champion (it's called artistic billiards in Europe), put on several free demonstrations of massé and stroke shots that dazzled onlookers.

Most of the tournament was dominated by the record-shattering performance of Ceulemans. He began with a 50–18 rout of Saad in 35 innings, followed by a 50–34 win over Torres in 32, and a 50–41 win over Doyharzabal in 33. And he was only getting warmed up! I arrived at the halfway point of his game with Legarda and was met in the exhibition room by pool champion "Champagne" Eddie Kelly, who was shaking his head in disbelief. He gave me the news that Ceulemans was leading 26–7 in only seven innings! I found a seat in the tournament room and made notes on the further progress of what was to be a record-tying game: 31–8 in 10 innings, 35–8 in 12; 47–11 in 18; and 50–12 in 20. The score sheet showed only five scoreless innings. His average of 2.5 tied his previous best world tournament game: 60 points in 24 innings.

As if that weren't enough, he came back with an even better game against Yoshihara. The fantastic Belgian ran 10 on the break at the start and 10-and-out at the end. It was 33–10 after 15 innings and 40–11 after 18. The game ended 50–12 in 19 innings, a new world tournament mark. Yoshihara, who is utterly impassive while playing and does not speak English, was almost effusive when leaving the arena, smiling, shrugging helplessly, and rolling his eyes at the sky. He had just seen God at work.

Ceulemans's last game in the round robin was against Zanetti, a handsome 25-year-old from Italy who took up three cushion only in recent years after becoming world class in balkline and one cushion. Ceulemans brushed him aside 50–30 in 27 innings, finishing his first six games with an unprecedented average of 1.807. That bettered the world record of 1.678 he set in 1978, the last time he played in Las Vegas. That man *loves* Las Vegas.

Or does he? By winning his bracket, Ceulemans advanced to play

Rico, the runner-up from the other seven-man flight. The loser would be relegated to playing for third and fourth place. Joining Ceulemans in the single-elimination was the runner-up from his flight, Zanetti, who had lost only to him and Yoshihara. The Japanese was denied a chance for the title by losing to Doyharzabal, Legarda, and Torres. Torres took third with his 3–3 record by virtue of his .967 average, better than Yoshihara's .935.

In the other bracket, the favorites were Blomdahl, who has eight tournament wins over Ceulemans and has been tagged by the 19-time world champion as a future title-holder, and the veteran Kobayashi. But Kobayashi was upset by Gilbert, and Blomdahl stumbled against Rico, so when the two met in the final round-robin game the loser would have two losses and would fall into third if Rico beat Gilbert. (Rico had lost only to Kobayashi and had tied Hallon.) As it turned out, Rico beat Gilbert 50–36, to reach the semifinals with Blomdahl, who beat Kobayashi 50–35.

The Americans, alas, played well but not well enough. U.S. champion Carlos Hallon lost an opening heartbreaker to Gilbert 50–48, tied Rico in his next game, beat Al Mashak, then suffered successive defeats by Blomdahl, Thieriaga, and Kobayashi. Gilbert, after dodging Hallon's bullet with the help of an 11 run, was upset by a man he thought he would beat, the unknown Thieriaga of Portugal, 50–40 in 48 innings. He came back with an impressive win over Kobayashi, 50–26 in 42, but his hopes of qualifying for the finals were dashed in his next game by Blomdahl, who beat him 50–27 in 36. He beat Al Mashak, but even a win against Rico in the final game wouldn't have been enough. It would, however, have put Kobayashi into the finals instead of Rico.

Torres did a little better in the other bracket. He began with an encouraging win over Yoshihara, a small man who uses a bridge between 10 and 15 inches long on almost every shot, and followed with another important win over Legarda, going out in only 39 innings. Then came losses to Ceulemans and Zanetti and a win over Saad. In his final game of the round robin, he had a slim chance of qualifying with a low-inning win over Doyharzabal, but he lost 50–42 in 45. His 3–3 record and average of .967 gave him third place in his bracket and the right to play Kobayashi for fifth and sixth place.

Nobody had been paying much attention to Rico after his early-round tie with Hallon and his wipeout by Kobayashi, 50–22. But at 9:30 P.M. on Saturday, May 17, there he was on table No. 1 taking on the invincible Ceulemans. Make that *almost* invincible. Nobody gave Rico a prayer, given the fantastic pace that Ceulemans was setting. Most of the game followed a script that has become common: a doomed world-class player struggles valiantly, averages over a point an inning, and gets crushed. In the 12th inning, Ceulemans came to the table leading 14–10 and ran 14, missing the 15th by a hair. It was 32–13 after 18 innings, when the scrappy Spaniard ran a three and a six to make it 36–22. When he trailed 44–25 after 28 turns, he came up with two, three, four, and one in successive innings to make it 48–35. The stage was set for one of the most electrifying runs in the history of the game.

The score sheet shows blanks for Ceulemans in six of his last nine innings, and several were shots that he usually makes with monotonous precision. Some say he eased up when the game passed 27 innings, which he needed to maintain his dizzying 1.8 average. Others say he got too interested in the game on the adjoining table between Blomdahl, who has become a thorn in the side for him, and Zanetti, a newcomer to world competition. Still others say he made a couple of questionable shot choices, perhaps in an effort to go out in a crowd-pleasing way. After all, at the end of his 30th turn he was leading 47–27 and hardly expected to *lose*. He needed three and Rico needed a doctor.

When Rico had 35 and began his stunning run, the tension in the hall began to build. The applause, polite after the first few points, rose as he reached the king row. When he had seven and trailed only 48–42 with the balls still in good position, Ceulemans's wife, Angel, sitting a few feet from her husband, began to pale and fidget, as did their close friend Steylarts. Ceulemans nodded silently, as if conceding that a miracle could be taking place. When Rico made the 10th and 11th points and trailed 48–46, Ceulemans briefly lowered his face into his hand. The balls were still in the open table, Rico was stroking quickly and confidently and had a great chance to make four more. It didn't seem fair, Ceulemans must have been thinking along with many in the audience, that an undefeated player scoring with unprecedented efficiency should be denied the world title on the basis of one run. But that is what was taking place. Rico scored the final points as if the balls were on strings and the spectators, already on their feet, exploded with applause and cheers.

Ceulemans, ever the gentleman, congratulated the victor and even managed a smile, but inside he was fuming, later vowing never again to play under such a format. Many of the fans in the bleachers, accustomed to complete round-robins for such important events, didn't realize that the single loss dropped the mighty champion into a playoff for third and fourth. It was the most stunning reversal imaginable and it took a while to sink in. Ceulemans was rolling over the opposition like a runaway locomotive toward what looked like his 20th world title. Then suddenly he was shunted onto a siding by a brilliant display of shotmaking by a player most Americans never heard of.

When the winning point was scored, someone behind me, no doubt thinking of Kareem Abdul Jabbar, Willie Shoemaker, and Jack Nicklaus, said excitedly: "It's the year of the old guy!" I turned around to see who it was. It was an old guy.

What Rico had accomplished was amazing. It is quite an accomplishment to beat Ceulemans under any conditions, but to do it in a game that eliminated him from title contention, to do it with a run of 15-and-out, and to do it in a world tournament when everybody in the house thought he couldn't—and thought he *shouldn't*—was nothing short of phenomenal.

The title game on Sunday between Rico and Blomdahl, who had gotten past Zanetti easily, 50–24 in 30 innings, was anticlimactic and almost dull—for a time. Blomdahl, tall, thin, and square-shouldered, has a quick, almost rushed style that fits his youth. In contrast, the short, serious Rico is placid and studious. When the game began, the two players must have remembered the recent European Championship, where they met twice. There the Swede edged the Spaniard 50–46 in the preliminaries, then came from far behind to beat him 50–48 in the title match. After trailing in the European Championship 10–27 after 14 innings and 25–41 after 31, Blomdahl caught fire and scored 25 points in 13 innings while Rico made only 7. So unnerved was Rico by the youngster's explosion that he missed a chance to run two to tie by hitting the end rail first on the break shot.

In Las Vegas it was almost the same scenario, but with the characters reversed. Blomdahl jumped out to leads of 13–2, 27–7, 33–11, and 37–13. When it was 41–25, the same score that had been reached in the European final, lightning struck Rico again and the magic returned. He ran a beautiful eight, then a few innings later a seven. At the end of 39 innings it was 46–44 Blomdahl, but the leader began to feel the heat and dogged a couple of shots, including a natural that fell two feet short. Rico kept scoring with nerveless efficiency, taking the game 50–46 and setting off the most memorable display of joy and emotion I have ever seen in a billiard room.

It was a jarring defeat for Blomdahl, who came so close to being the youngest three-cushion champion in history. But he will have dozens of additional chances, while Rico, at 55, had to strike when the iron was hot—and man, it was *hot*.

Rico, who plays at the beautiful Madrid Billiard Club in Spain, is not unknown in Europe, where he is respected as a dangerous if inconsistent foe. I first saw him in the 1974 world tournament in Antwerp, Belgium, where he finished seventh in a field of 12 and averaged .845. He has played many times in the European championship, finishing fourth in 1976 with an average of .934 and second in 1986 with an average of 1.027. According to Ben DeGraf of Holland, a top European sports journalist with a special interest in billiards, Rico's best tournament game is 60 points in 31 innings and his best run—in the Spanish championship—is 17. Before his electrifying run of 15-and-out against Ceulemans, the Belgian had beaten Rico 20 times in a row.

In the consolation games, Ceulemans beat Zanetti 50–36 in 28 innings for third place, Kobayashi beat Torres for fifth, Yoshihara beat Gilbert for seventh, Thieriaga beat Legarda for ninth, Doyharzabal beat Hallon for eleventh, and Saad beat Mashak for thirteenth.

One of the dignitaries on hand was Jay Bozeman of Vallejo, Calif., America's last link to the days of Willie Hoppe and Welker Cochran and the man Danny McGoorty called the best player who was never world champion. Ceulemans's 19-inning game reminded him of the time he made 41 points in 8 innings and then took 19 more innings to get to 50.

The tournament was a triumph for Jerry Karsh, president of the Billiard Federation of the U.S.A., and his international staff of 40 volunteers. Staging an event of this magnitude and importance requires a tremendous amount of work, and the task in 1986 was doubly difficult because of actions taken by backers of the proposed pro league. Karsh didn't know until just weeks before opening lag if his top stars, including Ceulemans, would show up. How he and his wife, Ann, kept their sanity, or even their composure, in the face of the billiard turmoil that was raging in Europe may never be known to historians. Rare for a billiard tournament was the profit shown. Expenses of $35,000 were more than offset by income of $37,000.

At the closing awards banquet, which featured music and dancing, A. E. Gagnaux, president of the World Union of Billiards, praised Karsh and his team for a well-organized, smoothly run event. He also defended the format, which had been criticized by some, for enabling a darkhorse like Rico to win. Everybody knows that Ceulemans is the best player, he stated, but it is not good for any sport if the best player or team always wins. The public roots for the underdog, is thrilled by impossible upsets, and is intrigued by the influence of luck and injustice. A full round-robin favors the best player, true, but it also results in a great many meaningless games. In billiards Ceulemans sometimes has round-robin tourneys locked up before the last round, or even the last two rounds, which takes the life out of what should be the most exciting phase. By switching to single elimination at the end, a final day of crucial matchups is guaranteed—which is especially important when television is involved.

The victory by Rico will have the effect of enlivening the games of Ceulemans for years to come. It will no longer be a foregone conclusion that he will win no matter how much better he is than his opponent nor how one-sided the score. It might even drive him to become a still more awesome billiard machine. And as for the underdogs, also-rans, and nobodies of the world, Avelino Rico has provided a wonderful demonstration that handicaps are sometimes not as impossible as they seem, that hope should never be abandoned, and that dogged persistence can eventually pay off in a big way.

The billiard gods are sometimes smiling, and one day they may smile at *you*.

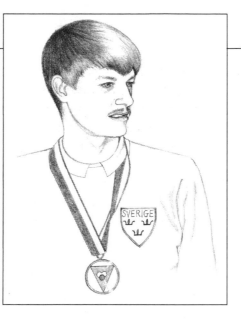

Dawn of the Blomdahl Era

RAYMOND CEULEMANS'S DOMINATION OF THREE-CUSHION BIL-liards had to end sometime, but after 25 years—from 1962 to 1987—it had begun to seem as though it would last forever. There have always been pretenders to the throne, especially in Europe and Japan, but the iron-willed Belgian's grip tightened as the years rolled on.

Finally there seems to be a successful usurper, a square-shouldered, straight-featured, fearless Swede named Torbjörn Blomdahl, who was born in 1962, the year before Ceulemans won his first world championship in three cushion. (Ceulemans was born in 1937).

That Ceulemans has lost his customary position atop the pyramid is not so much because his skills have declined—though after more than 100 national and international titles that could be expected—as it is sensational play of Blomdahl.

Blomdahl had remarkable success against Ceulemans right from the time he broke into the big time in 1981 while still a teenager. He won four of their first eleven meetings, then won five straight to emerge as a nemesis for the world champion and heir apparent to his title.

A harbinger of the future was an amazing game they played in the 1985 European team championship. Playing to 50 points, Ceulemans had 43 points at the end of 19 innings, an average of 2.263, which is terrific even for him. Blomdahl, though, had 50 points for an average of 2.631.

At the world tournament at the Tropicana Hotel in Las Vegas in 1986, the two finished behind upstart Avelino Rico of Spain. Despite finishing third, Ceulemans showed that he was far from finished by averaging 1.746, which topped the record of 1.678 he set in the same city in 1978.

Later in the year they parted company. Blomdahl continued playing for the Union Mondial Billard (UMB), while Ceulemans jumped to a new professional league called the World Billiard Association (BWA). Blomdahl won his first world championship by winning the UMB's ultimate event in Cairo, Egypt, topping Frank Torres of the United States in his final match. The pro group staged "Grand Prix" events in France, Belgium, Germany, and the Netherlands. By winning one and finishing second three times, Ceulemans was declared the first world's professional champion since the days of Willie Hoppe, edging Japan's Nobuake Kobayashi. Ceulemans's prize winnings were $51,450 for the season.

Blomdahl joined the pro tour in 1987 and finished second to Ceulemans despite averaging 1.503 for the five ranking tournaments. He won the world title the following year and finished second to Belgium's Ludo Dielis in 1989, with Ceulemans third. In 1990 Ceulemans reasserted himself, taking the crown and relegating Blomdahl to second place. In 1991 it was Blomdahl on top again, with Ceulemans second. An exciting development for Americans in 1991 was the strong play of the fast-rising Sang Chun Lee, former Korean champion, who now is a naturalized United States citizen and owner of a billiard room in New York City. The 38-year-old Sang Lee finished the year ranked fourth in the world and in the Berlin leg of the pro tour finished first, beating Ceulemans in the final game.

A surprising twist is that one of the five BWA tournaments in early 1989 and the UMB's 1989 European championship as well were won by 49-year-old Lennart Blomdahl, Torbjörn's father!

If the Ceulemans era is not over, it has at least been interrupted. It's hard to imagine anyone matching his record of 20 world three-cushion titles, but Torbjörn Blomdahl at least has a shot at it.

Ceulemans is a powerful player and a menacing presence at the table, and it will be interesting to see if he can maintain the intensity, desire, and concentration that were among the reasons he stayed on top so long. Perhaps Blomdahl, who has a restless and impatient style, will go on to other things. (To pool, for example. He has entered several world-class nine-ball tournaments in Europe and finished among the leaders every time.)

The three-cushion matches between Blomdahl and Ceulemans in the next few years promise to be epic and fascinating struggles, like surf pounding a rockbound shore. Several of the matches will take place in the United States. The BWA has added Las Vegas to its list of Grand Prix sites. In Las Vegas, Ceulemans always seems to be at his superhuman best.

It should be remembered that Ceulemans is a master not just of three cushion but also of straight billiards, balkline, and one cushion, disciplines that Blomdahl set aside in his breathtaking rush to the three-cushion peak. Anyone who has seen Ceulemans give an exhibition of stroke and massé shots knows that if he ever retires from three-cushion competition and takes up what the Europeans call artistic billiards, he could well win world titles and set records in that form of the game as well.

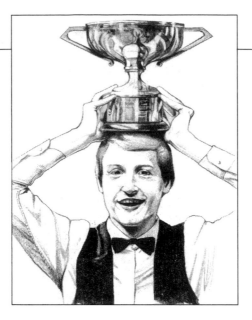

The Boom You
Hear Is Snooker

IN TERMS OF TELEVISION COVERAGE, WHAT IS THE BIGGEST AN-
nual sporting event in the world? No, it's not the Rose Bowl, the Super
Bowl, the World Series, the Wimbledon Tennis Tournament, or the
Grand National Steeplechase. The answer would astound the average
American sportswriter or sportscaster: The Embassy World Professional
Snooker Tournament in Sheffield, England.

Never has a mere game been given such massive television
coverage. BBC-TV (British Broadcasting Company) assigns 256 people
to the event for 17 days and broadcasts more than 100 hours of *live*
action . . . if you can call it action. I was in England in 1984 to cover
the tournament and was amazed at the attention such a slow-paced
game is given by the media. As an American accustomed to a daily dose
of electronic violence, I found it eerie to watch the tube in the home
of a London friend and see minute after long minute spent on two men
exchanging carefully thought-out safeties. The cameras studied their
faces, their hands, and the position of the balls, and in contrast to sports

coverage in the United States, the commentators generally kept their mouths shut unless they had something useful to say.

Before boarding a train to the tournament site in Sheffield, an industrial city north of London, I asked my friend's grey-haired grandmother why she glued herself to the screen. This was a woman who had never played the game and had only a vague understanding of the rules. "Because it is so serene," she replied. "No killing or bombs or car chases. Sometimes I turn off the sound and just watch the picture. The young men are handsome and the colors are restful."

Whatever her reasons for watching, she is not alone; the tournament attracts more than half of the British television audience. So handsome are the young men and so well dressed that more than 50 percent of the viewers are female.

Except for a few morning sessions early in the tournament, the 1,000-seat arena was filled three times a day. (By my own estimate, about a third of the paid admissions were female.) Without spending a penny on advertising, the promoters sold 30,000 tickets by mail a month in advance.

While snooker has been around for 100 years in England and its former colonies worldwide, it hasn't always been so popular. The boom started in the late 1970s when corporations, finally persuaded by the impressive ratings for televised snooker, began sponsoring tournaments and the BBC began covering them. Since then the number of major events, the yearly prize money totals, the number of televised hours, the size of the audience, the fame and fortune of the players all have climbed together to breathtaking heights.

In 1974, England's four television channel's broadcast about 20 hours of snooker a year. Starting in the 1978–79 season the incredible boom began and the yearly hours advanced to 55, then to 88, then to 120, 180, and 240. In the 1987–88 season, snooker players, snooker fans, and those who simply like to see well-dressed men bending over tables were able to enjoy 357 hours of snooker on television.

In 1976–77 there were only two major tournaments, in 1981–82 there were eight, and in 1983–84 there were twelve. Now, with the addition of a foreign tour that includes Canada, Indonesia, Hong Kong, Australia, and New Zealand, countries where snooker is the game of choice, there are 24.

Yearly prize fund totals have grown from $30,000 in 1977–78 to $185,000 in 1979–80, $530,000 in 1981–82, and a stunning $870,000 in 1983–84. For 1990 hang on to your hat—the total will be around $3,500,000, about 10 percent of which will come from the foreign tour.

The climax of snooker season, the Embassy World Tournament, has been the catalyst. When Embassy (part of Imperial Tobacco Limited) first sponsored the tournament in 1976, there were 28 entrants fighting for $15,000. In 1984 there were 94 players and a record-breaking prize fund of $260,000. The winner got $59,000, the runner-up $30,000. Prizes ranged downward to $3,000 for the 16 first-round losers. One can only cry at the memory of the late, great Joe Davis, who won the world championship in 1927 and received the grand total of £6, 10*s* . . . about $14.

For winning the 1989 Embassy, Steve Davis (pictured in the drawing on page 218) took $168,000 from the prize fund of $840,000. His prize winnings for the season totaled just over $1 million.

Embassy is getting its money's worth, for direct advertising of its products is banned on British television. While I was in the country there was a letter to the editor of the *London Times* complaining about the way tobacco, whiskey, and beer companies were using snooker tournaments to escape restrictions on television advertising.

For the top players, prize winnings are just the beginning. Exhibitions, lessons, and especially endorsements are a bigger part of the pie. Steve Davis, only 26 years old in 1984, won more than $130,000 in each of the previous two years and made at least $800,000 a year in other snooker-related income. He is treated like a major media star, as in fact he is, and is one of the best-known people in Great Britain. He has written two popular books on the game (with a ghostwriter's help), is a frequent subject of magazine and newspaper pieces, and has his own fan club, complete with Steve Davis pens, key chains, posters, videotapes, and photographs. There is even a Steve Davis newsletter to keep the teenage groupies happy.

All of the top players are treated like celebrities. Not even rock music stars get more attention. Of course rock stars, or celebrities in any part of show business or politics, aren't on television 320 hours a year.

I realized I was in wonderland when I first arrived at the tournament site, Sheffield's Crucible Theatre. At the stage door was a crowd of about 100 people, mostly but by no means entirely youngsters, hoping to get a glimpse of one of the players. In the lobby was Willie Thorne, the number 18 seed, trapped by autograph seekers. A man in a red coat whose photo I couldn't find in the tournament program was also signing autographs—later I learned he was one of the referees. Even the refs are stars! (So thoroughly organized is snooker in Britain that it takes about ten years for a referee to work his way up to a world tournament. A players' committee has the final word on acceptability.)

Snooker is played with 21 balls on a table measuring 6-by-12-feet, though in the United States a common size is 5 by 10. The pocket entrances are narrow and rounded so that it takes extreme accuracy to make a ball that is close to the rail. The game is played by alternately pocketing the fifteen red balls and the six numbered balls (two through seven); the reds stay down, the numbers are respotted. When the reds are gone, the numbers are pocketed in order and stay down. The highest possible run is 147, which results from making all fifteen red balls, which score one each, a 7-ball following each red, then all the numbered balls, which count their face value. (Davis has done it during a match on live television.) Points are also scored when a player's opponent fails to hit the required ball, which makes safety play a direct offensive weapon.

The game is closer to straight pool than nine ball in that it is seldom necessary to shoot hard or send the cueball very far. Pinpoint accuracy is essential, which rules out the use of very much sidespin. Good snooker players resort most often to high, low, and centerball, as sidespin has too great an effect on accuracy. As in one-pocket, you have to have the discipline and knowledge to resist some open shots and go for a safety instead. To play at the top level you need to be a superb shotmaker, you need excellent speed control, and you need to be able to judge follow, draw, and deadball shots to within a hair's breadth.

Professional snooker is governed by the World Professional Billiards and Snooker Association. Some of the WPBSA tournaments are invitational, some are "open." Americans who are thinking of taking a shot at the tempting prize money should know that by "open" the WPBSA means "open to WPBSA members." To become a member you have to apply and state your qualifications. (The address is 77 Charlemont Road, West Bromwich, West Midlands, B71 3DY, England.) There are presently 125 members of the association. The only American members are Jim Rempe and Steve Mizerak, who have tried to qualify several times for the final 32 at Sheffield with no success. The snooker champions are good at what they do, make no mistake about it.

The top American players would have a hard time beating any of the top 50 snooker players, in the opinion of Clive Everton, editor of *Snooker Scene.* By the same token the best snooker players have no chance against the best Americans in nine ball or straight pool. The games and the equipment are just too different.

American players would also have a hard time adjusting to the attention of the fans and the press. It seems, in fact, that some of the British players aren't adjusting to it too well, either. Players used to obscurity and living on a shoestring suddenly find themselves with more money and notoriety than they know how to handle. A magazine article that appeared while I was in England began: "However dignified the players may seem on television, however rarefied the atmosphere—don't be fooled. The behaviour of many of the world's top professional snooker players makes music's pop stars seem like a pack of goody-goody choir boys."

The author found a disgruntled ex-wife of one of the players and quoted her as follows: "They drink like fish. They are nothing but a bunch of spoiled brats. Everyone keeps telling them how great they are and they believe it. They're drunk with all the television coverage.

"It's heartbreaking to see what snooker success has done to a lot of them. I've seen them come along as nice, open, honest, friendly kids and within a couple of years they're ruined. They do it in front of your eyes. They become takers. They grab everything on offer and a lot of them become big-headed and demand to have all sorts of things done for them.

"Apart from snooker, all that most of them think about is getting drunk and sleeping with girls. The only other thing many of them think about is gambling. They don't do anything else but lie around to recover.

"They have great success with girls. After the evening's play, the lads go off to nightclubs. They don't have to try very hard because the girls seem to go into heat the moment they see a snooker player. It is quite incredible. The girls just leave their husbands and boyfriends, come straight across and crawl all over them. The guys don't even have to chat them up.

"My husband had to choose between snooker and me, and I lost."

The 1984 Embassy World Professional Snooker Championship, a 32-man single elimination, was held from April 21 to May 7. The top 16 seeds were exempt from qualifying; the next 16 had to play knockout matches against the 16 survivors of a two-week qualifying tournament among the other 62 players. Half of those ranked 17th to 32nd were eliminated in the matches against the challengers. Among the survivors was 70-year-old Fred Davis, the formerly unbeatable champion who is now ranked 28th. Newcomers making it to the Crucible included 19-year-old John Parrot and 20-year-old Neal Foulds.

The tournament was superbly managed. The WPBSA had 38 people on the scene, Embassy (which staffed a press room where the telephones, food, drinks, and closed-circuit TV were free day and night) had 20 people, and the BBC had 256. What makes this the biggest televised sporting event in the world is that the BBC must provide a full crew of 80 technicians three shifts a day for 17 days. Nothing else in sports comes close, except the Olympics.

Games were played on only two tables, and after the introduction of the players and referees a screen was lowered between them so that players on one table would not be distracted by what was happening on the other. Two cameras on dollies were trained on each table plus a portable camera. Two more cameras were set up in the interview room. Every shot taken during the entire tournament was either shown live or taped.

A first for the 1984 tournament was a glassed-in soundproof enclosure close to the tables for photographers. In the lobby of the area was a booth for placing bets, which is legal in Britain. Bets could be placed on players to win the tournament (Davis was so heavily favored that the odds on him were 12 to 11) or on the outcome of any given match. Odds were sometimes changed while a match was in progress. Coral, the licensed company that handles snooker betting, estimated that it would handle about $2,500,000 in snooker wagers in 1984, compared to a mere $30,000 in 1978.

In the first round the matches consisted of a race to 10 frames (games); in the next two rounds it was a race to 13; in the semifinals a race to 16. The final match was a race to 18. Since a frame of snooker takes from 10 to 60 minutes, even a first-round match can take from four to six hours. Here is a major difference in approach between Britain and the United States. Over there the players are expected to fight it out over two, three, or even four long sessions before a winner is decided. The schedule broke the early matches in two and allowed a total of eight hours to reach a decision. Twenty years ago, when fewer players were competing, races to 40 were common. A single-elimination format is not quite so unfair when matches are played at such length.

The big news in the first round was the defeat by young Neal Foulds of the mercurial Alex "Hurricane" Higgins, a cocky hustler type who fought his way up from the slums of Belfast to win world championships in 1972 and 1982. He is a great popular favorite because of his image as a blue-collar scrapper challenging the privileged upper classes and his unpredictable behavior. The early departure of Higgins took a lot of color out of the tournament.

One of the Canadian entrants in 1984 was Mario Morra, who told me he has played a lot of nine ball and prefers it to snooker because it isn't as tedious. He is concentrating on snooker, though, because that's where the money is. Because of the scarcity of tournaments and sponsors in Canada, he has moved to England to be close to the action. The cue he uses for snooker is typical: 54 inches long, 17 ounces in weight, and 10 millimeters in diameter at the tip, with a black ferrule. He made an interesting technical point during our conversation: Even though a snooker table is bigger than a pool table and the pockets are smaller, it's easier to bank a ball in snooker because of the blunt rubber. Pool rubber has a knife-edged nose that makes it more sensitive to speed.

In the first round of 1984's Embassy, Morra lost to countryman Cliff Thorburn, 10–3.

Another highlight of the first round was the defeat by young John Parrot of lady's man Tony Knowles, whose sexual boasting in the morning paper had turned much of the audience against him.

The audience, by the way, was the best-behaved I have ever seen. It was strange to see 1,000 people freeze in perfect silence when a player was aiming. I didn't even hear any coughing. The politeness and self-control of the spectators reminded me of what Milton Berle used to say when faced with a crowd that wasn't responding to his jokes: "What is this, an audience or an oil painting?"

In the second round, Steve Davis hardly needed the allotted three sessions to get past John Spencer, 13 frames to 5.

In the quarter finals, Davis, a cool scoring machine if there ever was one, opened with a run of 94 against Terry Griffiths and went on to take the match, 13–10.

The semifinal matches were the best of 31, which required four sessions. Steve Davis ground out a relentless if not exciting win over Dennis Taylor, 16–9. The other match, between Jimmy White of Tooting (only in England could there be a place with such a name) and Canada's Kirk Stevens, was memorable for White's upset stomach. He twice had to run from the arena to throw up, once in the middle of an 85-point run. Rumor had it that he had chosen inappropriate food and drink to celebrate his 22nd birthday the night before. Trailing 12–10 at the end of the third session, White rallied in the fourth to win 16–14.

The final match between the mechanical Davis and the excitable White looked like it was going to be a rout for the machine. After the first two sessions Davis led 12–4 and needed only six more frames to win. On the second day, White started with a run of 119 and went on to take the third session 7–1, making the overall score 13–11 Davis.

A Sordid Snooker Saga

SNOOKER'S IMAGE WAS SET BACK IN 1984 BY THE DARKLY HANDSOME Tony Knowles. The second-ranked player in the world at the time, Knowles is especially popular with the girls. He gets mail by the sackful from groupies, some with return train tickets and provocative photos. Knowles does nothing to counteract the playboy image that Britain's so-called gutter press presents of him.

On the contrary, he encourages it. The April 24, 1984, edition of the sleazy *Sun* featured Knowles on the front page in a tuxedo with one arm around a cue and the other around a blonde wearing little beside mesh stockings. Inside he is shown lying beside her on a snooker table under the headline: "Why Girls Call Me the Hottest Pot in Snooker." The article states that Knowles "knows all about scores—off the table as well as on. The hottest shot in the game pockets more birds than balls. Girls fall over themselves to get within groping distance. They climb through windows, bribe officials, shower him with presents, and pretend to be his sister, just to get close."

"The only thing I offer them," Knowles is quoted as saying, "is a lift home. The only meal I ever buy them is breakfast. I rate girls on a scale of two— those who say yes and those who say no. I don't meet many who say no."

The *Sun* series on Knowles ran three consecutive days coinciding with the start of the Embassy tournament. On the fourth day—the morning after Knowles was unexpectedly knocked out of the tournament by John Parrot— the *Sun* blasted its star in a feature titled "Tony: You're a Lousy Lover," authored by Knowles's ex-girlfriend.

The appearance of such sensational articles, even in a rag that specializes in them (every day the paper runs a photo of a bare-breasted woman on page 3), was an embarrassment to tournament officials. You can't stop a tabloid from making up quotes, but in this case Knowles didn't disown the remarks attributed to him . . . and he obviously cooperated by posing for the photos. (Knowles reportedly received more than $30,000 from the *Sun* for his cooperation.) Not amused, the WPBSA fined Knowles $6,500—by far the largest fine ever levied by the WPBSA—for his lack of taste and for his seeming indifference to the game's image.

Clive Everton in *Snooker Scene* wrote that White was "roared on by a crowd which rose to his bravery against apparently hopeless odds. Not since Ray Reardon beat Eddie Charlton from six down with nine to go in the 1975 final had the game's greatest occasion seen such a dramatic reversal."

In the final session, Davis pulled ahead 16–12, but White kept the crowd electrified by winning the next three frames to pull to within one. When it was 17–16 Davis, both players began to crack a bit under the pressure, missing shots they normally would make, but in the end it was Davis who steadied himself to win the 34th frame, thus taking the match 18–16.

The champion is the exact opposite of the hell-raising, skirt-chasing stereotype that the London scandal sheets portray as the typical snooker star. He is calm, clean-cut, clean-living, polite, well-spoken, and always immaculately groomed. He credits his mum and dad with his success. He would be perfect as a Boy Scout leader or rector in the Church of England. His spotless, squeaky-clean image, in fact, is one reason he makes so much on endorsements. He'll never embarrass a sponsor by climbing onto a snooker table to pose with a half-draped sex kitten.

If you ever get to England, don't fail to take in at least one day of a snooker tournament featuring Steve Davis. You'll not only see a man who has become one of the country's most famous landmarks, you'll see a scoring machine of withering efficiency. Perfection, that's what Steve Davis has dedicated himself to, and he's almost there.

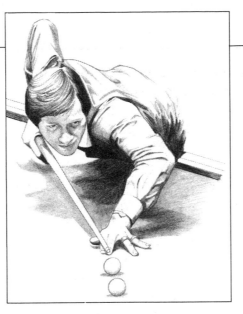

Hurricane Higgins,
Britain's Bad Boy

I N 1972, BOBBY FISCHER PUT CHESS ON THE FRONT PAGES OF newspapers around the world. His outrageous antics during the title match against Russia's Boris Spassky shattered the stereotype of chess as a game for old coots who couldn't remember whose move it was and changed it forever into a spectator sport with big prizes for the winners.

Jimmy Connors and John McEnroe did something similar for tennis. Their boorishness, temper tantrums, and contempt for upper-crust decorum were denounced by everybody, but by turning tennis into bloody warfare, complete with screams, curses, and thrusting fists, they made it fascinating to people outside the game. The result was soaring television ratings and a shower of money for all concerned.

The ratings for big-time golf are slipping, and why? Because the players are as much fun as cloistered monks. The game needs another Tommy Bolt, who at any minute might blow his cork and wrap his niblick around the nearest caddy. Golf tournaments today are like FBI picnics.

Which brings me to Alex "Hurricane" Higgins, the bad boy of professional snooker. He makes Fischer, Connors, McEnroe, and Bolt look like partners for bridge. Hurricane is almost too mild a nickname. When he's blowing gale force, he'll tell the most distinguished snooker official in the world to take a flying love-act at a revolving pastry. When he throws a party in his hotel room, it's something the other guests, the hotel staff, and the local police talk about for the rest of their lives.

I've met him twice, and both times he was friendly and a model of decorum. "He's Dr. Jekyll and Mr. Hyde," one British snooker watcher told me, referring to Stevenson's tale of split personality. "Unfortunately, he's 90 percent Hyde." I've seen only the 10 percent.

His bouts with the bottle, and his exuberant style of living in general, have cost him a truckload of money. He makes $100,000 a year in prize money, which isn't that much if you're a party animal, but almost nothing in endorsements. He presents the wrong image. Squeaky-clean Steve Davis, on the other hand, No. 1-rated snooker player in the world, makes around a million a year in prizes and triple that in endorsements. (Only his accountant knows for sure.) What corporate sponsor would take a chance on Alex Higgins? He might throw a fit and moon a major client.

Alex is a brawler from Belfast, Northern Ireland, and was born there in 1949. He liked playing money matches—hustling, we call it here—playing the horses, and having a good time. *The Hustler* was his favorite movie. When he reached the finals of the 1972 world snooker tournament at the tender age of 23, he was the people's choice, a roughneck from the wrong side of the tracks who had battled his way to the top without the benefit of teachers, schooling, or coaches. He had no permanent home. He had, by his own account, recently lived in a row of abandoned houses in Blackburn, staying one jump ahead of the bulldozer and wrecking ball; in one week he had five addresses: 9, 11, 13, 15, and 17 Ebony Street.

His opponent in 1972 was defending world champion John Spencer, a well-mannered 38-year-old much in the mold of the staid snooker establishment. Alex, on the other hand, with his nicotine-stained fingers and bloodshot eyes, looked like a juvenile delinquent . . . a disgrace to the dignity of the grand old game, in the opinion of the dusty guardians of propriety. As Gordon Burn writes in his book *Pocket Money*, "He is a product of the Jampot, the billiard hall in the Donegal Road area of

Belfast, where he grew up on Mars bars, Coke, and Players Extra. He's raw, abrasive, and contemptuous of authority of any kind. He believes he's the best player who has ever played the game and, unbelievable in a world where restraint and discretion have long been bywords, keeps going round saying that he is."

After two sessions a day for six days, Alex wins the deciding frame and is the youngest world snooker champion in history. It is like the barbarians sacking Rome, and it is witnessed by one of the biggest and most boisterous crowds in snooker's history. "The trophy is presented," Burn writes, "by one of the old-timers, a former champion who, in common with many of those present, does his best to put a brave face on what he expects could turn out to be a catastrophe."

A party in his hotel that night leaves his room soaked with beer and littered with bottles and overturned chairs. "He will celebrate his title," Burn tells us, "by travelling to Australia, where he will be thrown out of one club for rubbishing a senior player and out of a hotel for demolishing his room. He will move on to India, where he will be escorted onto a return flight less than 24 hours after arriving for getting drunk, stripping, and sticking his hand up an old man's dhoti."

Needless to say, the British newspapers, several of which are the trashiest in the world, had a field day with such an outlandish character. Alex's shenanigans were headlines and he dragged snooker with him into the limelight.

In every tournament, the match everybody wanted to see was Davis against Higgins, icy control against total chaos, nerves of steel versus hot blood.

Total prize money for the 1972 tournament was £800 . . . about $1,400. Alex's first-prize check was for £480. But snooker was being talked about and noticed in England and four years later the prize fund for the world tournament had grown to $15,000 and began to more than double every year. When television took over in a big way in the early 1980s, the game and the rewards exploded upward.

Most analysts expected the Hurricane to blow himself out quickly because of his life-style, but he showed remarkable endurance and in 1982 stunned the snooker establishment again by winning his second world title, this time snagging a check worth almost $40,000. He was married by then with two toddlers, and when he held the winner's trophy over his head and faced the cheering crowd he was openly crying.

Success didn't calm him down. He continued to be mainly interested in a good time, not in pleasing the snooker authorities. At one tournament he failed to show up for an awards ceremony, a snub to the officials that fellow Irishman Dennis Taylor excused by saying: "Alex went to Belfast to launch a ship and won't let go of the bottle."

I first met him in 1984 at the Embassy World Tournament, held every year in a 1,000-seat theater in Sheffield called the Crucible. After winning in 1982 and losing in the semifinals the year before, he was bounced out in the first round in 1984 by 20-year-old Neal Foulds. Nevertheless, Higgins, after taking a half-hour to recover from the shock, came to the press room and chatted amiably with reporters.

He was cocky even in defeat, and in response to my questions about pool and three-cushion billiards, claimed to be adept at those games as well. He went so far as to offer to play any American any game for any amount of money, and to show he was serious he gave me his address and phone number. All he asked was a month to practice with someone who knew the game. I should have tested his bravado by trying to set something up, but I had trouble believing he was serious. His contempt for pool as a game that was too easy was almost a joke.

His hard drinking and flashpoint temper finally began to take their toll. In 1986 his world ranking had slipped to ninth, and for a dispute after a tournament game in Preston, in which he bumped a referee in anger, he was fined £12,000 and banned for five tournaments.

I went on vacation in England and Scotland in September 1988, and while I hadn't intended to do any reporting, the game of snooker there is hard to avoid. In my hotel room the first night in London, I flipped on the telly and saw Steve Davis saying a good word for a certain brand of baked beans. Later I saw an absolutely amazing commercial— a group of young men are playing snooker in a pub, a player takes a shot and causes the ball to fly through the air toward the bartender, who calmly catches it. Doesn't seem like much until you realize that the entire thing was filmed *underwater!*

A snooker tournament was under way at Stoke, near Liverpool. My schedule didn't allow me to attend, though I watched hour-long summaries every night on the tube. Steve Davis beat Jimmy White in the final, setting a world record by running 100 points or more in three successive games. Snooker's imperturbable scoring machine admitted that it was the best he ever played.

Alex Higgins had been eliminated in the first round, as had a number of other notable players, and was participating in a "satellite" tournament in Glasgow, Scotland. One Saturday afternoon I managed to find the tournament site, Marco's Leisure Centre, a two-story brick building that contained a full health club—swimming pool, racquetball courts, spa, and weight room—as well as 40 6-by-12-foot snooker tables.

Even though there were no facilities for spectators other than a few chairs along one wall, the players were shooting for £25,000 in prize money. First prize was £5,000 (about $8,800). In addition to Higgins, the event attracted such players as John Spencer, Canada's Bill Werbeniuk (a whale of a man who claims he drinks beer on doctor's orders), Graham Miles, and South Africa's Peter Francisco, all high on the world ranking list. Alex's world ranking had sunk to 17th, making him the second seed in the tournament behind Francisco.

To be ranked 17th, incidentally, is a whole lot worse than 16th. The top 16 are seeded into the world tournament as well as into the British Masters.

So far out of favor had Alex fallen that only four people took chairs next to his table. It was a race to five. Alex seemed nervous at the start, but was clearly the superior player and gradually pulled ahead despite errors on both sides. He is slightly built and probably weighs no more than 140 pounds. Nervous energy flows through him and he rarely is completely still. He has a square face that flickers with emotions he can't conceal. He sat next to me a time or two when his opponent, Mike Fisher, was shooting, muttering about how much he hated the table. "Every shot is an adventure," he said at one point.

In the second frame he wanted something to settle his nerves. "I need a bit of the hair of the dog," he whispered to me. "Would you mind going out to the bar and getting me a lager with lemon? I'll pay you later."

The brew seemed to help him, and in the final two games he played some brilliant snooker, getting a run of 85 in one and 50 and out in the other, finishing with a flashy length-of-the-table bank on the final black. He took the match 5–2.

He didn't pay me later, but he did something better; he asked me to join him for a drink. He couldn't have been nicer. There is something appealing and heart-wrenching about the guy. He's divorced now. He had an agent, but sacked him. He owned a house, but sold it. "It's embarrassing for me to play in a tournament like this," he confided, "but I need the readies . . . you know, the bucks, the dollars."

He explained that his cue was giving him some trouble. Knowing that the table wouldn't be of world-championship caliber and that he would have to shoot harder than he normally would, he added a half-ounce to the butt by drilling a small hole in the end and inserting a piece of metal. That upset the balance and was bothering him.

He sipped a screwdriver. Nearby Werbeniuk was tossing down

beer after beer. Several players were sitting in the bar with their one-piece cues in long cases.

Alex didn't remember our meeting in 1984. He guessed, in fact, that I made cues. When I reminded him of his challenge to play any American any game for any amount of money with just a month to practice, he wasn't quite as cocky as before. He changed the terms. Now he wants *six months* to prepare, and he wants as a training partner one of the particular game's top ten players.

"If I did that," he said, "nobody would have much chance." Under those terms, the chance of arranging a match are nil.

Does he practice snooker? "After winning the world title in 1982, I thought I didn't have to practice. Then my marriage went sour and my game went downhill. Now before a tournament I practice 25 hours a week."

Peter Francisco came by and Alex introduced me to him, remembering my name. That impressed me. Most top players are too caught up with themselves to remember names.

He won me over with his openness and friendliness. It breaks my heart to see such talent being held back by whatever demons control him. But he isn't the type to seek help, which suggests that he is on an irreversible slide toward oblivion, taking his talent with him.

In the days that followed I spent time in Wales and Ireland. I bought a paper every day to see how Alex was doing. He came within an eyelash of winning the Glasgow tournament. In the deciding game of the final match, he watched the surprising Gary Wilkinson (ranked 102) run 56 and out to win on the final ball.

A bombshell was in the next day's paper under a headline that read: "Higgins on Carpet Again."

Alex Higgins must face a disciplinary committee set up by the World Professional Billiards and Snooker Association at Bristol. Higgins was reported to the WPBSA for his behaviour following the final of the Professional Player's Tournament at Marco's Lesiure Centre, Glasgow, on Monday night.

The twice former world champion was furious at being asked by officials to give a urine sample after losing 5–4 to Gary Wilkinson. He did eventually give a sample in a public toilet in front of photographers.

How can you not love a guy like that? Good luck, Alex, wherever you are. I, for one, am rooting for you.

(Alex escaped with a reprimand. In January of 1989 he broke his foot in a fall from a first-floor window at his lady-friend's flat, but won the Irish championship hopping on one leg. By the end of 1989 he had managed to lift his ranking to 16th from a low of 24th.)

Walter Lindrum, Legend from Down Under

Walter Lindrum, Billiards Phenomenon, by Andrew Ricketts. Hardcover, 1983, 192 pages, 49 photos, $24.00. Published by Walter Lindrum Publishing Syndicate, Australia. (To order, make check out to "M. P. Giuliano for Walter Lindrum Syndicate" and mail to Walter Lindrum Publishing Syndicate, c/o M. P. Giuliano, P.O. Box 158, Nunawading, Victoria, 3131 Australia.)

WHO WAS THE GREATEST WIELDER OF A CUE IN ALL OF HUMAN history? The answer depends on where the question is asked. In the United States, Willie Hoppe, Welker Cochran, Willie Mosconi, and Ralph Greenleaf would be nominated; in Europe, Raymond Ceulemans; in South America, votes would be cast for Ezequiel Navarra; in Japan there are those who favor old-timers like Yamada and Matsuyama; in Britain, Steve Davis. The problem, of course, is that the game has to be specified. Cochran, Hoppe, Yamada, and Matsuyama played billiards on the pocketless table, as do Ceulemans and Navarra; Steve Davis is a snooker expert; Greenleaf played pool, as does Mosconi.

In Australia there would be no argument at all: everybody would vote for Walter Lindrum. Walter Lindrum was world champion in a form of the game called English billiards. It is played on a 6 by 12 "snooker" table with three balls, and points are scored by pocketing one of the two object balls (potting), caroming the cueball off the two object balls (a cannon), or by deliberately scratching off one of the object balls (a hazard). It was the main game played in England and its former colonies until the 1930s, when snooker gradually took over as the favored style of play.

Lindrum was so far above the competition that the rules were changed in an effort to slow him down. He responded by retiring after only two years as the official world champion, 1933 and 1934. He had little interest in snooker, which he considered a much inferior game, and nobody was able to persuade him to play competitively again. In snooker exhibitions during World War II, however, he had many runs of over 100.

Walter Lindrum's grandfather was a billiard room owner and so was his father. In Andrew Ricketts's well-written and deeply researched book on Lindrum, it is reported that on the night Walter was born in 1898, his father was playing billiards for money in the goldfields of Western Australia. Not world class as a player himself, the father set out to make his other son, Fred, world champion, imposing a rigorous regimen of practice sessions on him that kids today wouldn't stand for. Fred won the Australian championship 27 times, but couldn't handle the champions from England, so the father turned to Fred's younger brother, Walter, a less colorful but more systematic player. Walter responded brilliantly, getting so good that he almost killed the game single-handedly.

During the 1929–30 season in England, Ricketts points out, he had 67 runs of more than 1,000 points, more than any other player has made in a lifetime. The great Joe Davis was smashed, and in a two-week match with Lindrum accepted a 7,000-point spot and still lost. In a match with Davis in 1932 the Aussie ran 4,137, a record that still stands.

I found one of the most interesting features of this book the references to the practice methods the father set out for his two sons. For example, for six months Walter was allowed to use only one ball. When he could leave it with precision on any part of the table, a second ball was added. One drill he had to practice for hours at a time was shooting the cueball from a distance of about two feet into a ball frozen on the rail, making the cueball rebound softly to its starting point.

Walter Lindrum, Billiards Phenomenon is beautifully bound and printed in hardcover on high-quality paper, contains 49 photos, has

192 pages, and is indexed. American readers will find it slightly disorienting because of the narrow focus on a game they've never seen played. There is an assumption in these pages that English billiards and snooker are the only cue games there are. Surely a book that sets out to establish that a certain individual was "the greatest billiard player of all time" should at least *mention* people like Ceulemans, Greenleaf, Mosconi, and Schaefer. (Hoppe and Cochran, whose first name is incorrectly given as Walter, are mentioned, but only in passing.) Once you get used to the insular point of view, though, and words like potting, hazards, and cannons, you'll have a good read.

Congratulations to Andrew Ricketts for a fine piece of scholarship. Somebody should do a book like this on Ralph Greenleaf.

Robert Craven's
Billiard Bibliography

Billiards, Bowling, Table Tennis, Pinball, and Video Games: A Bibliographic Guide, by Robert Craven. Hardcover, 1984, 179 pages, $29.95. Published by Greenwood Press, P.O. Box 5007, Westport, Conn. (When ordering by mail, add $1.00 for postage.)

ALMOST EVERY PLAYER OWNS AT LEAST ONE BOOK ON THE game; most own several. Serious players wishing to leave no stone unturned in their efforts to improve buy every book they can get their hands on. Then there are the collectors who want not only the latest titles but the earliest ones as well and aren't particularly interested in whether or not the book is "good" or "bad"; more important than the contents are the book's condition and scarcity.

All lovers of pool and billiards should applaud the appearance of Robert Craven's bibliography of billiard books, but collectors should go outside right now and turn handsprings of joy. Never before have those interested in the literature of the game had a deeply researched list like this, which contains the basic facts on practically every title published in English in the last 200 years. Book collectors and historians now have a good idea of the scope and contents of their field of interest—previously everybody was groping in the dark, wondering what the limits were.

Have you ever emerged from a second-hand bookstore with a 1913 edition of *Daly's Billiard Book* or an 1891 edition of *Modern Billiards* and wondered how many editions were published and when and where and by whom? Look it up in Craven. Or just browse and be amazed by the richness and diversity of the game's printed legacy—the book contains 618 listings in the billiard section. (Other sections are devoted to the table games given in the title.)

The book measures 6¼ by 9½ inches, has 179 pages overall, and is well-bound in hardcover. Because of the limited audience for a scholarly work like this, the price is relatively steep: $29.95. Only 50 pages are devoted to pool and billiard listings, but those 50 pages are priceless to researchers, bibliophiles, and miscellaneous students of the game. Three additional pages are devoted to an interesting review of billiard publishing from its beginnings in the late 1700s to the present.

The pool and billiard listings are subdivided into Pre–1800; 1800–99; 1900–39; 1940–69; 1970–82; selected foreign-language books; newspapers and magazines; and selected articles. The book is fully indexed and includes a prefatory article on sports reference works as well as an explanation of the author's research methods.

Robert Craven is Associate Professor of English at New Hampshire College in Manchester. I hope the publication of this book helps him in his academic career because I can't imagine it making him rich in the marketplace.

About the Author

Robert Byrne has been involved in cue games for over thirty years as a player, tournament promoter, teacher, collector of memorabilia, journalist, and author.

As a pool player he has won tournaments in eight-ball, nine-ball, straight pool, and snooker. In three-cushion billiards he has twice finished among the top four in the United States National Championship.

His four books on the games of pool and billiards have been widely praised for their accuracy, clarity, and style, and his two videotapes are considered among the best instructional tapes ever made on any game or sport.

He is also the author of six novels, four of which have been selected by Reader's Digest Condensed Books.

Robert Byrne lives in Iowa.

Also
published by
Harcourt Brace & Company

and available as Harvest/Harcourt Brace paperbacks

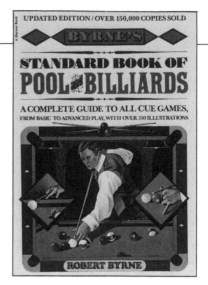

UPDATED EDITION / OVER 150,000 COPIES SOLD

BYRNE'S

STANDARD BOOK OF
POOL and BILLIARDS

A COMPLETE GUIDE TO ALL CUE GAMES,
FROM BASIC TO ADVANCED PLAY, WITH OVER 350 ILLUSTRATIONS

ROBERT BYRNE

"*The* definitive work on pool and billiards."

The National Billiard News

"No doubt about it—this is the most comprehensive and finest dia-grammed exposition ever devised of the 'art and science' of pool and three-cushion billiards. . . . Be warned: The book, which is for both novices and the very advanced, can be ruinous to family harmony. Also health: You may never see the sun again." *Village Voice*

"Thorough without being overly complex and writing in a delightful style, Byrne takes the reader from basics to most advanced shots."

Los Angeles Times

"The book I've been waiting for. The artwork, the writing, the organization, the scope . . . everything is absolutely tops. A great book by the perfect author." Dorothy Wise, Five-time U.S. Women's Pool Champion

"A tremendous work. It far surpasses anything else on the market, and should belong in every billiard player's library."

Al Gilbert, Seven-time U.S. Billiards Champion

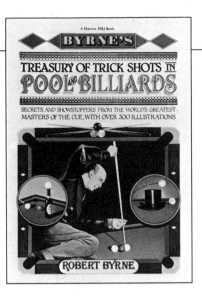

"The most comprehensive collection of knowledge and facts I have ever read between two covers. It will be an outstanding addition to any collection of pool and billiards books for years to come. I was fascinated by it."   Ray Abrams, Copublisher, *The National Billiard News*

"The most complete book on the subject I have ever come across. I especially like the historical notes."

Jimmy Caras, Four-time World Champion and author
of *Trick and Fancy Shots in Pocket Billiards Made Easy*

"Bob Byrne has provided exciting new shots and ideas to go with dozens of rediscovered classics and familiar standards, and this book deserves to stand beside *Byrne's Standard Book of Pool and Billiards* on any player's bookshelf. It puts at your fingertips techniques and ideas that would normally take years to acquire."

Paul Gerni, Seven-time World Champion, Trick and Fancy Shots

"In my forty years in this game I've never met anyone with Bob Byrne's contacts with top players around the world, his knowledge of the technique and history of the game, and his writing ability. You can get happily lost in these pages for days on end."

E. J. Pilotte, former President, Billiard Federation of the U.S.A.